Conservative
Infertility Management

REPRODUCTIVE MEDICINE & ASSISTED REPRODUCTIVE
TECHNIQUES SERIES

Series Editors

David K Gardner DPhil
Colorado Center for Reproductive Medicine, Englewood, CO, USA

Jan Gerris MD PhD
Professor of Gynecology, University Hospital Ghent, Ghent, Belgium

Zeev Shoham MD
Director, Infertility Unit, Kaplan Hospital, Rehovot, Israel

Forthcoming Titles

Conservative Infertility Management

Christoph Keck MD
Department of Gynecological Endocrinology
and Reproductive Medicine
PAN-Hospital
Cologne
Germany

Clemens B Tempfer MD
Department of Obstetrics and Gynecology
University of Vienna
Vienna
Austria

Jean-Noel Hugues MD
Reproductive Medicine Unit
Department of Obstetrics and Gynecology
Jean Verdier Hospital
Paris
France

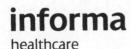

informa
healthcare

First published in 2007 by Informa Healthcare, Telephone House, 69-77 Paul Street, London EC2A 4LQ, UK.

Simultaneously published in the USA by Informa Healthcare, 52 Vanderbilt Avenue, 7th Floor, New York, NY 10017, USA.

Informa Healthcare is a trading division of Informa UK Ltd. Registered Office: 37–41 Mortimer Street, London W1T 3JH, UK. Registered in England and Wales number 1072954.

A CIP record for this book is available from the British Library.

ISBN-13: 9780415384513

Orders may be sent to: Informa Healthcare, Sheepen Place, Colchester, Essex CO3 3LP, UK
Telephone: +44 (0)20 7017 5540
Email: CSDhealthcarebooks@informa.com
Website: http://informahealthcarebooks.com/

For corporate sales please contact: CorporateBooksIHC@informa.com

For foreign rights please contact: RightsIHC@informa.com

For reprint permissions please contact: PermissionsIHC@informa.com

Contents

Contents

Preface

It is estimated that in developed countries approximately 15% of couples suffer from infertility. Since Louise Brown was born in 1978 as the first baby after successful IVF treatment, dramatic changes have taken place in this field of research. Not only have the overall pregnancy rates for assisted reproductive techniques (ART) significantly improved, but also new techniques, such as ICSI, TESE, PGD, etc. have become standard treatment options. If such a spectacular development takes place within a relatively short period of time there is always a certain risk that these advanced techniques will be applied without fully exploiting the possibilities of a more conservative approach. In clinical practice we sometimes see patients undergoing IVF or ICSI treatment without having been investigated properly and without having been counseled about any other treatment options.

In recent literature and most of the textbooks published in our field over the past decade there is a similar trend: there are numerous textbooks on the latest advances in ART and far fewer books and papers on conservative treatment options. This book has been written to fill a gap and to provide the reader with a comprehensive overview of diagnostic and conservative therapeutic approaches for infertility treatment. The most common diseases in reproductive endocrinology such as endometriosis or polycystic ovary syndrome are discussed, as well as new drugs for ovulation induction or ovarian stimulation.

We hope that this book is useful for both general gynecologists and for IVF specialists in order to broaden their therapeutic spectrum. Furthermore, we sincerely hope that it helps patients to receive the treatment they need in order to fulfil their wish for a child.

Christoph Keck
Clemens B Tempfer
Jean-Noel Hugues

Color plates

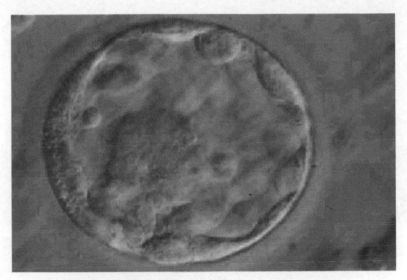

Plate 1 (Figure 2.13)   The human blastocyst

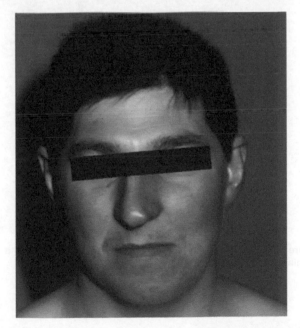

Plate 2 (Figure 3.2)   A 45-year-old patient with Klinefelter's syndrome and characteristic straight frontal hairline and lacking beard growth

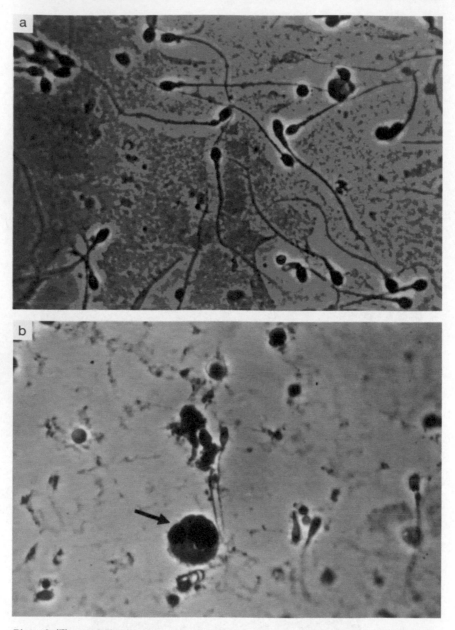

Plate 3 (Figure 3.5) (a) Normal sperm morphology; (b) detection of a leukocyte by peroxidase staining;

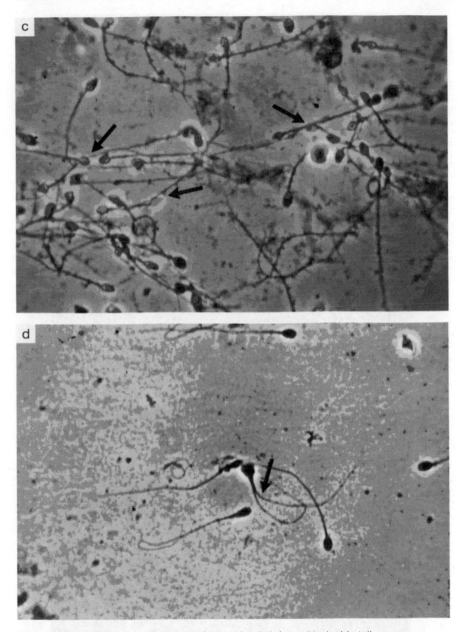

Plate 3 (Figure 3.5)   (c) acrosome defects; (d) tail defect with double tail

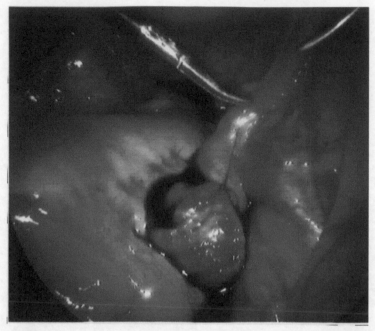

Plate 4 (Figure 3.15) Laparoscopic assessment of tubal patency: extrusion of the methylene blue solution through the distal end of the right tube is clearly visible

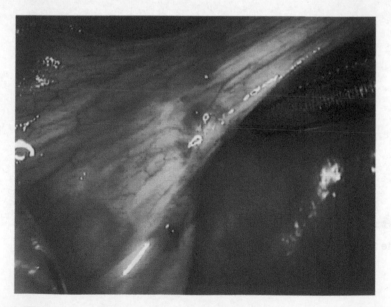

Plate 5 (Figure 4.1) Minimal endometriosis at the uterine ligaments in a 23-year-old patient without clinical symptoms

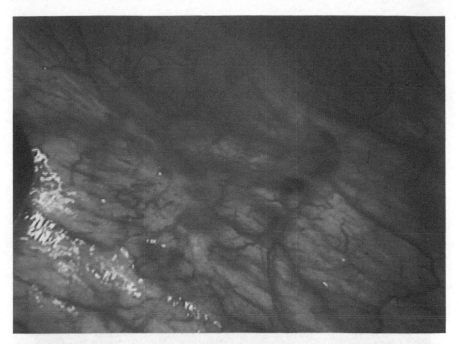

Plate 6 (Figure 4.2) Minimal endometriosis at the pelvic wall in a 30-year-old patient without symptoms

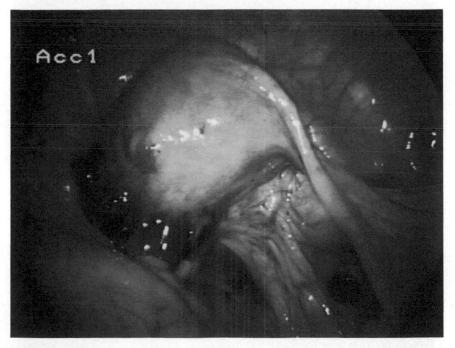

Plate 7 (Figure 4.3) Massive endometriosis in a 24-year-old patient with adhesions between uterus, sigma, left adnexes and pelvic wall

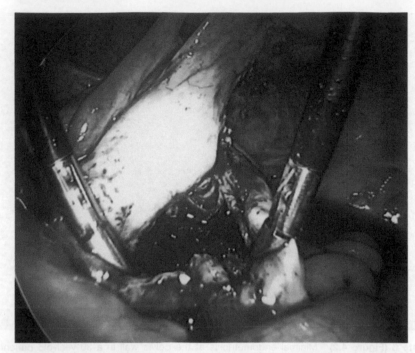

Plate 8 (Figure 4.4)   Chocolate cyst of the left ovary. Surgical removal of the cyst

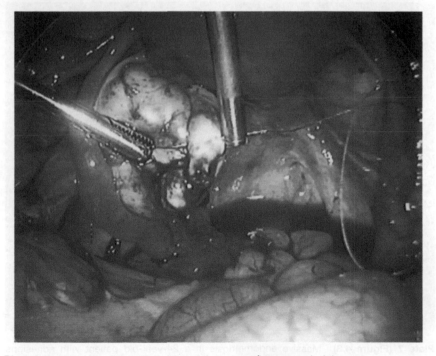

Plate 9 (Figure 4.5)   Reconfiguration of the ovary after removal of the cyst

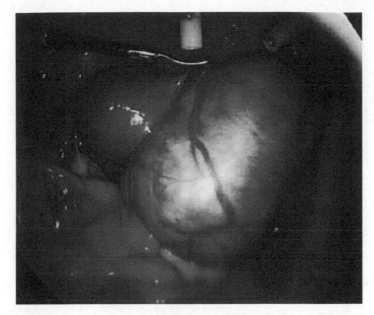

Plate 10 (Figure 4.7) Subserous fibroid in a 28-year-old woman. Infertility for 3 years. Diameter of fibroid: 8 cm

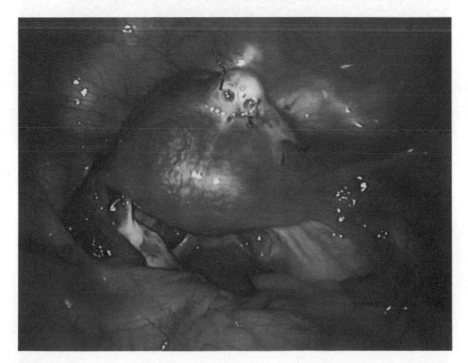

Plate 11 (Figure 4.8) Situs after laparoscopic removal of the fibroid

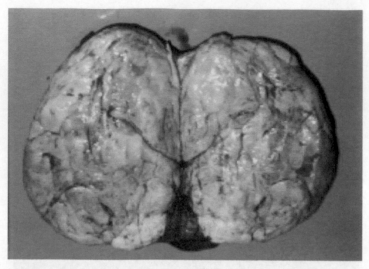

Plate 12 (Figure 4.9) Typical macroscopic aspect of fibroid morphology

Plate 13 (Figure 4.10) Typical microscopic picture of a fibroid:
* muscle fibers form vortex-like structures
* ovoid or nearly rectangular nuclei
* sometimes nuclei arranged in palisades
* varying amount of collagen fibers

1

Epidemiology of infertility

DEFINITION

Infertility and related terms need to be defined, because in the literature they are sometimes used interchangeably.

- In demography, the terms fertility and infertility refer to reproductive performance in a purely descriptive manner. They are used whether or not there was a live birth during a certain period of time, and do not take into account whether or not the couple wished to conceive. The capacity of a couple to produce a live birth is called fecundity or ability to conceive. The complete lack of that capacity is called infecundity or sterility.

- In contrast, in reproductive medicine, the term infertility is used for couples who have had unprotected, regular intercourse for a certain period of time and who have failed to achieve a pregnancy. In addition, the term subfertility is used to define any form or grade of reduced fertility in couples unsuccessfully trying to conceive. As the definition of subfertility and its prevalence are linked, it seems essential to provide valuable parameters such as time to pregnancy (TTP) and cumulative probabilities of conception (CPC). Thus, suitable thresholds can be used to determine the prevalence of grades of subfertility and, in cases where the prognosis is poor, may be used as indicators for the timing of routine investigations and for starting treatment[1].

PREVALENCE

Infertility is currently defined as 1 year of unwanted non-conception with unprotected intercourse in the fertile phase of the menstrual cycle[2].

1

In a recent study of 363 women using natural family planning methods to conceive[3], the estimated CPC at 1, 3, 6 and 12 cycles were 38, 68, 81 and 92%, respectively. As expected, CPC declined with age.

Humans are not fertile mammals. Indeed, if we consider the monthly fecundity rates (MFR), the average estimate is only 20%[4]. Evers and Te Velde[5] developed a mathematical model to show the extent to which different MFRs arise in the general population (Table 1.1). It appears that, between fertile couples (MFR 100%) and infertile couples (MFR 0%), there is a continuous distribution of MFRs from 0% to about 60%. Table 1.1 shows that about 93% of normally fertile couples will conceive within 1 year and that 11% of severely subfertile couples will also achieve a pregnancy.

Nevertheless, other authors[3] suggested that the question of subfertility must be raised after six cycles of unprotected intercourse without conception, regardless of age, because most women < 30 years of age should have conceived by that time. Furthermore, treatment such as *in vitro* fertilization (IVF) also seems justified in women over the age of 35 years, because their chance of live birth decreases rapidly. It may thus be proposed that the first infertility investigations should be performed after six cycles with timed intercourse. Thus, a prognosis statement and a detailed grading of subfertility, ranging from 60% to nearly 0% chance of spontaneous conception, is possible[6]. In cases with a good prognosis, couples should be encouraged to wait, with self-monitoring of the menstrual cycle (cervical mucus observation; basal body temperature chart) to identify peak fertility and to improve pregnancy prospects. In cases with a poor prognosis, assisted reproductive treatment should be discussed. This applies only in cases with poor prognosis as regards tubal patency and male infertility.

Table 1.1 Hypothetical model of cumulative monthly fecundity rates (MFR) (%). Adapted from reference 2, with permission of Elsevier

		Cumulative pregnancy rate after			
Category	MFR	6 months	12 months	24 months	60 months
'Superfertility'	60	100	—	—	—
Normal fertility	20	74	93	100	—
Moderate subfertility	5	26	46	71	95
Severe subfertility	1	6	11	21	45
Infertility	0	0	0	0	0

Finally, it should also be pointed out that the prevalence of infertility is different in different areas around the world[7]. In most developing countries, the proportion of permanently infertile women is low compared with that reported in developed countries. This may be due to marriage and pregnancy occurring at a younger age than in developed countries. The picture changes when one considers secondary infertility. The high secondary infertility rates in developing countries are likely to be explained by the high incidence of sexually transmitted infections and medical interventions under unhygienic conditions, particularly postpartum.

CAUSES OF INFERTILITY AND PERSPECTIVE

A balanced management of reduced fertility requires appropriate timing of infertility investigations and appropriate timing of starting treatment, to avoid both over- and undertreatment.

A routine work-up screens for causes of infertility and is used to predict prognosis both with and without treatment. As shown in Table 1.2, five distinct subsets of subfertility catagories are usually described. A couple can have more than one cause of infertility between them and all factors of subfertility must be taken into account when considering the chances of conception.

Table 1.2 Distribution of causes of subfertility in primary, secondary and tertiary care. Adapted from reference 2 with permission

	Primary care (%)* (n = 726)	Secondary care (%) (n = 708)	Tertiary care (%) (n = 2198)
Cause of subfertility			
Male factor	20	26	24
Ovulation	24	21	18
Cervical mucus	15	9	—
Tuboperitoneal†	11	20	30
Unexplained‡	30	25	3
Other	—	—	3

*Data correct for multiple causes; †includes moderate and severe endometriosis; ‡includes minimum and mild endometriosis

Male factor

A male factor is the dominant cause of subfertility in 20–26% of couples[8–10]. Semen analysis is the main method of male fertility assessment. Although azoospermia is an undisputed cause of male infertility, male subfertility is much more difficult to diagnose. World Health Organization (WHO) criteria stated that a man can be judged normally fertile if his sperm count is 20×10^6/ml, progressive motility > 50% and normal morphology > 30%[11]. In addition, two studies reported the relation between semen variables and the achievement of pregnancy within 12 months in order to define cut-off values below which fertility is judged impaired[12,13]. They reported remarkably similar cut-off values: 14.3×10^6/ml and 13.5×10^6/ml for sperm concentration, 28 and 32% for progressive motility and 5 and 9% for normal sperm morphology (Kruger criteria), respectively.

Ovulation dysfunctions

The only absolute proof of ovulation is pregnancy, because other tests cannot exactly assess the frequency and consequences of ovulation disturbances. A regular menstrual cycle and adequate progesterone concentrations or endometrial biopsy results cannot verify ovulation. Conversely, an irregular menstrual cycle cannot prove anovulation but is an indicator that further tests should be done. Most disturbances can be detected through measurement of follicle stimulating hormone (FSH), estradiol and prolactin plasma concentrations and by ovarian ultrasound assessment.

Spermatozoa–mucus interaction defects

Cervical hostility has been considered responsible for subfertility in 9–15% of couples by some authors[8,9], but others have denied its existence[10]. The debate on the predictive value of the postcoital test is ongoing. Griffith and Grimes[14] reported that the sensitivity of the test ranged from 9 to 71%, the specificity from 62 to 100%, the predictive value of an abnormal test from 56 to 100% and the predictive value of a normal test from 25 to 75%. However, many issues should be addressed, for example the proper timing by ultrasound and the cut-off values for positivity. Furthermore, as reported by Glazener et al.[15], it is likely that the postcoital test is an effective predictor of conception only if defined female causes of subfertility are absent and duration of infertility is less than 3 years. Whether the postcoital test should

Table 1.3 Hysterosalpingography and laparoscopy for prediction of fertility outcome. Adapted from reference 16, with permission

| | Laparoscopy | | |
Hysterosalpingography	No occlusion	One tube occluded	Both tubes occluded
No occlusion	50/450 (11%)	0/24 (0%)	0/12 (0%)
One tube occluded	6/73 (8%)	3/26 (12%)	0/15 (0%)
Both tubes occluded	7/81 (9%)	2/44 (5%)	2/69 (3%)

Data are number of treatment-dependent intrauterine pregnancies/total number of patients (3-year cumulative pregnancy rate), according to type of tubal occlusion diagnosed at laparoscopy or hysterosalpingography

be an integral component of the routine fertility work-up is still a matter of debate. It is not commonly performed by physicians in many developed countries and, surprisingly, a positive postcoital test is not usually required to classify infertility as unexplained. The question of whether or not the postcoital test is helpful in identifying patients who would benefit from intrauterine insemination (IUI) needs to be discussed.

Tuboperitoneal disorders

Post-infectious tubal damage, tubal obstruction, hydrosalpinx, pelvic adhesions or endometriosis are the cause of subfertility in about 11–30% of couples, with an increased prevalence from a primary-care to a tertiary-care population. The woman's history and physical examination as well as a positive chlamydial antibody test can alert physicians to potential tuboperitoneal disorders. Mol et al.[16] compared the predictive value of hysterosalpingography and laparoscopy. As shown in Table 1.3, laparoscopy is able to predict pregnancy more accurately but is not the gold standard for diagnosis of fertility impairment related to tuboperitoneal disorders.

Unexplained infertility

According to previous reports[8–10], infertility seems to remain unexplained in 25–30% of fully investigated couples. However, it is quite evident that the proportion of couples with unexplained infertility decreases as the number of available diagnostic tests increases. As reported by Taylor and Collins[17], the prevalence of unexplained infertility decreased from 22% in studies published before 1960 to 14% in studies published after 1980, attesting to the key role of the thoroughness of the investigation. Moreover, the duration of infertility is essential. Indeed, the residual likelihood of spontaneous pregnancy in untreated couples with unexplained infertility fell from 40% after 3 years to 20% after 5 years[17].

As the cause of infertility is unexplained, treatment options are empirical. IUI associated with ovarian stimulation is usually the first-line therapy and improves the rate of pregnancy. While more demanding, IVF is usually recommended after failure of four cycles with IUI. One of the rationales to proceed to IVF is to control the ability of the sperm to fertilize. Nevertheless, it should be kept in mind that a spontaneous pregnancy rate of 5–9% per 12 months in patients on a waiting list for IVF has been reported[18]. Patients with minimal or mild endometriosis should be considered as suffering from unexplained infertility because the overall spontaneous pregnancy rate in eight trials (28%) did not differ significantly from that reported in unexplained infertility (33%)[2].

CONSEQUENCES – STRATEGY

The assessment of subfertility factors allows us to predict the chance of a couple conceiving naturally. It also provides useful information for counseling couples in the choice of treatment. The cost-effectiveness and the safety of conventional treatments also need to be considered. Beyond this, the question is whether or not the couple should be referred for assisted reproduction. This is a challenging issue that will be covered in the following chapters.

REFERENCES

1. Gnoth C, Godehardt E, Frank-Herrmann P, et al. Definition and prevalence of subfertility and infertility. Hum Reprod 2005; 20: 1144–7
2. Evers JL. Female subfertility. Lancet 2002; 360: 151–9
3. Gnoth C, Frank-Herrmann P, Freundl G, et al. Time to pregnancy: results of the German prospective study and impact on the management of infertility. Hum Reprod 2003; 18: 1959–66

4. Leridon H, Spira A. Problems in measuring the effectiveness of infertility therapy. Fertil Steril 1984; 41: 580–6
5. Evers JL, Te Velde ER. Vruchtbaarheidsstoornissen. In Heineman MJ, Bleker OP, Evers JL, Heintz AP, eds. Obstetrie en Gynaecologie, de voortplanting van de mens. Maarssen: Elsevier Science, 2001: 435–71
6. Habbema JDF, Collins J, Leridon H, et al. Towards less confusing terminology in reproductive medicine: a proposal. Hum Reprod 2004; 19: 1497–501
7. Lunenfeld B, Van Steirteghem A, on behalf of all participants. Infertility in the third millenium: implications for individual, family and society. Condensed meeting report from the Bertarelli Foundation's second global conference. Hum Reprod Update 2004; 10: 317–26
8. Hull MG, Glazener CM, Kelly NJ, et al. Population study of causes, treatment, and outcome of infertility. Br Med J (Clin Res Ed) 1985; 291: 1693–7
9. Snick HK, Snick TS, Evers JL, et al. The spontaneous pregnancy prognosis in untreated subfertile couples: the Walcheren primary care study. Hum Reprod 1997; 12: 1582–8
10. Collins JA, Burrows EA, Willan AE. The prognosis for live birth among untreated infertile couples. Fertil Steril 1995; 64: 22–8
11. World Health Organization. Laboratory Manual for the Examination of Human Semen and Semen–cervical Mucus Interaction. Cambridge: Cambridge University Press, 1987
12. Ombelet W, Bosmans E, Janssen M, et al. Semen parameters in a fertile versus subfertile population: a need for change in the interpretation of semen testing. Hum Reprod 1997; 12: 987–93
13. Guzick DS, Overstreet JW, Factor-Litvak P, et al. Sperm morphology, motility, and concentration in fertile and infertile men. N Engl J Med 2001; 345: 1388–93
14. Griffith CS, Grimes DA. The validity of the postcoital test. Am J Obstet Gynecol 1990; 162: 615–20
15. Glazener CM, Ford WC, Hull MG. The prognostic power of the post-coital test for natural conception depends on duration of infertility. Hum Reprod 2000; 15: 1953–7
16. Mol BW, Collins JA, Burrows EA, et al. Comparison of hysterosalpingography and laparoscopy in predicting fertility outcome. Hum Reprod 1999; 14: 1237–42
17. Taylor PJ, Collins JA. Unexplained Infertility. New York: Oxford University Press, 1992: 153–69
18. Evers JL, de Haas HW, Land JA, et al. Treatment-independent pregnancy rate in patients with severe reproductive disorders. Hum Reprod 1998; 13: 1206–9

2

Physiology

ANATOMICAL BASIS

The ovaries are located on the reverse side of the plica lata and are connected to the uterus by the utero-ovarian ligament (ligamentum ovarii proprium). The utero-ovarian ligament contains blood vessels originating in the ascending branch of the uterine artery. The ovaries are primarily perfused by the ovarian artery stemming from the aorta and passing through the ovarian suspensory ligament (ligamentum suspensorium ovarii). Blood leaves the ovaries primarily via the ovarian vein, which is also within the ovarian suspensory ligament (Figure 2.1).

At the onset of puberty, there are approximately 400 000 primordial follicles and single follicles in all stages of maturity in the ovary. Oocytes contained in the primordial follicles migrate out of the extragenital structures of the celomic epithelium into the stroma of the primary bipotent gonads as oogonia during embryonic development. These then divide further mitotically (Figure 2.2).

Development of the primordial follicle into the primary follicle is indicated by the appearance of the basement membrane. The germ cells in the primary follicle remain in the diplotene stage until ovulation, that is, with a diploid chromosome complement. Therefore, the second meiotic division of the female germ cell is completed only shortly before the fusion of egg and sperm.

Primordial follicles are found predominantly in the ovarian cortex. The primordial follicle consists of an oocyte surrounded by a layer of flat follicular epithelial cells, which are in turn surrounded by thecal cells. The primary follicle is differentiated from the primordial follicle by the enlargement of the oocyte, which is now surrounded by a basal membrane and cubic follicular epithelial cells (Figure 2.3). Next steps in follicular development involve the secondary and tertiary follicle. Development from primordial

9

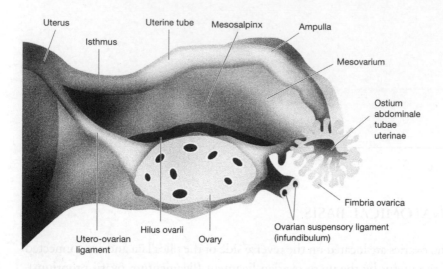

Figure 2.1 Anatomy of the female reproductive organs

follicle to the tertiary follicle usually takes 3 months. This development, until the stage of the mature Graafian follicle, is characterized by a proliferation of granulosa cells.

PARACRINE AND AUTOCRINE REGULATION

Cyclic ovarian function – entailing follicle maturation, ovulation, corpus luteum development and luteolysis – is regulated by the hypothalamic–pituitary system as well as by intraovarian mechanisms[1]. Hypothalamus, pituitary and ovary are thereby in dynamic interaction. Gonadotropin releasing hormone (GnRH) is synthesized in hypothalamic nuclei and reaches the anterior pituitary via the pituitary portal circulation. There, GnRH binds to specific receptors and induces expression and secretion of luteinizing hormone (LH) and follicle stimulating hormone (FSH). The release of the gonadotropin hormones is therefore GnRH-dependent and occurs in a pulsatile manner approximately every 90 minutes[2] (Figure 2.4).

The regulatory mechanisms behind pulsatile GnRH release remain unclear. Besides the sex steroids, which exert a regulatory influence on the function of GnRH-producing nerve cells, catecholamines and endogenous opiates are also involved in the regulation of GnRH secretion (Figure 2.5).

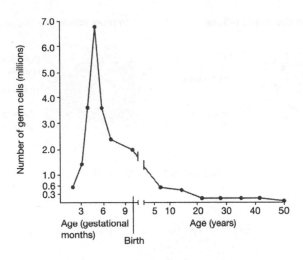

Figure 2.2   Number of germ cells throughout female life

THE OVARIAN CYCLE

At the beginning of the ovarian cycle or even before this, a number of follicles mature under the influence of FSH and most reach the antral follicle stage (Figure 2.6).

Of this cohort of maturing follicles, only one usually attains dominance. The mechanisms underlying the selection of the dominant follicle are unknown. It is thought that high intrafollicular estradiol levels represent a selection advantage by increasing sensitivity to FSH. Selection of the dominant follicle occurs approximately 6 days before ovulation. The remaining follicles in the cohort undergo atresia. The dominant follicle proceeds to develop into the so-called Graafian follicle. The Graafian follicle is morphologically characterized by a cystic structure approximately 2 cm in diameter and by a multilayer avascular follicular epithelial layer. The follicular epithelial cells make up the cumulus oophorus, which surrounds the oocyte (Figure 2.3).

APOPTOSIS IN THE OVARY

It is estimated that less than 1% of all follicles reach the stage of the Graafian follicle, with 99% of follicles degenerating by apoptosis. Programmed cell

a

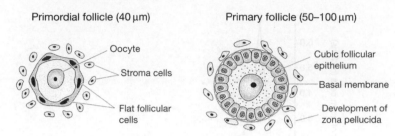

Primordial follicle (40 µm)

Oocyte

Stroma cells

Flat follicular cells

Primary follicle (50–100 µm)

Cubic follicular epithelium

Basal membrane

Development of zona pellucida

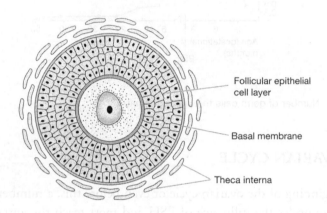

Secondary follicle (200 µm)

Follicular epithelial cell layer

Basal membrane

Theca interna

b

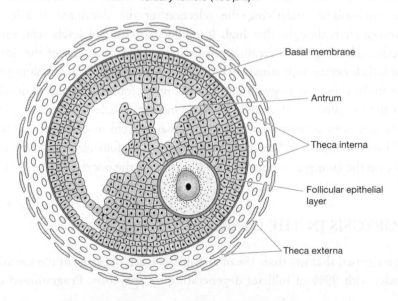

Tertiary follicle (400 µm)

Basal membrane

Antrum

Theca interna

Follicular epithelial layer

Theca externa

c

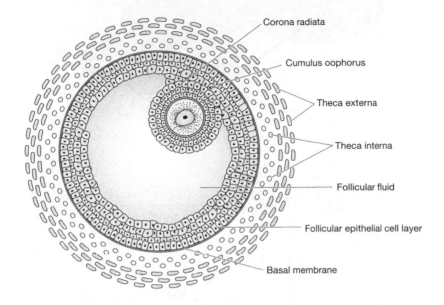

Mature tertiary follicle (Graafian follicle), up to 25 mm

Corona radiata

Cumulus oophorus

Theca externa

Theca interna

Follicular fluid

Follicular epithelial cell layer

Basal membrane

Figure 2.3   (a–c) Stages of follicle development with follicle diameters

death is an energy-dependent process accompanied by DNA degradation[4]. Apoptosis is initiated by activation of calcium-dependent endonucleases and finished by phagocytosis. In addition to an adequate FSH level, survival of a follicle also depends on growth factors such as epidermal growth factor (EGF), transforming growth factor β (TGF-β), basic fibroblast growth factor (bFGF), insulin-like growth factor (IGF-I) and estrogens[5]. The apoptosis-inhibiting effects of the growth factors EGF, TGF-β and bFGF are presumably mediated by tyrosine kinase (Figure 2.7).

OOCYTE MATURATION

As long as the oocyte remains within the follicle it remains diploid, so meiosis has not been completed. The second meiotic division is initiated and completed immediately after release of the egg from the follicle. Suspension of the egg in its diploid stage is regulated by intrafollicular substances, which

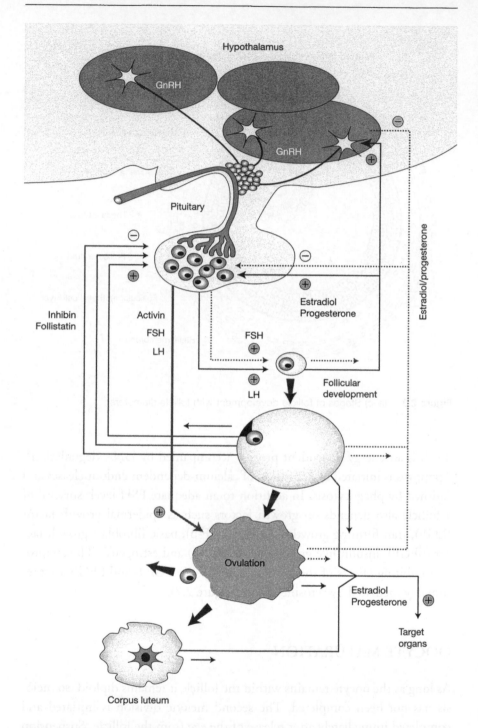

Figure 2.4 Interaction between hypothalamus, pituitary and ovary. Representation of the negative and positive feedback mechanisms

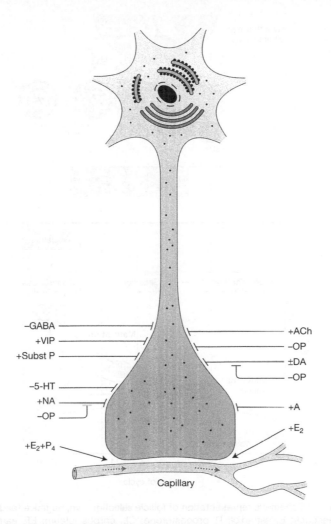

Figure 2.5 Inhibitory or stimulating influences on the function of GnRH neurons. GABA, gamma-aminobutyric acid; VIP, vasoactive polypeptide; 5-HT, 5-hydroxytryptamine; NA, noradrenaline (norepinephrine); OP, opioids; ACh, acetylcholine; DA, dopamine; A, adrenaline (epinephrine); E_2, estradiol; P_4, progesterone. Adapted from reference 3

prevent meiosis. Among these is oocyte maturation inhibitor (OMI), which is a product of the follicular epithelial cells. OMI is a polypeptide with a molecular mass of approximately 2 kDa. The exact chemical structure of OMI is not known. Also unknown is whether substances such as inhibin, activin and the various growth factors prevent oocyte maturation until LH-induced ovulation. Research is ongoing to unravel the puzzle of meiosis arrest.

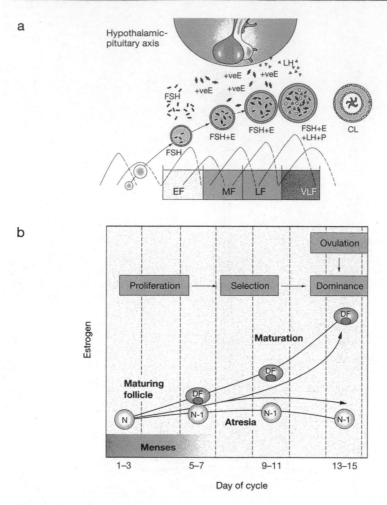

Figure 2.6 (a) Schematic representation of follicle selection. -ve, negative feedback; +ve, positive feedback; E, estradiol; P, progesterone; CL, corpus luteum; EF, early follicular maturation phase; MF/LF, mid/late follicular maturation phase; VLF, very late phase. (b) Schematic representation of follicular maturation and selection of the dominant follicle. N, number of maturing follicles. Adapted from reference 3

OVULATION

The dominant follicle begins to express LH receptors on the follicular granulosa cells prior to ovulation. This process is FSH-dependent. Estradiol secretion is simultaneously increased, which causes an increase in pituitary synthesis and storage of LH. An LH peak occurs by means of a positive feedback mechanism. The mean interval between maximal estrogen production

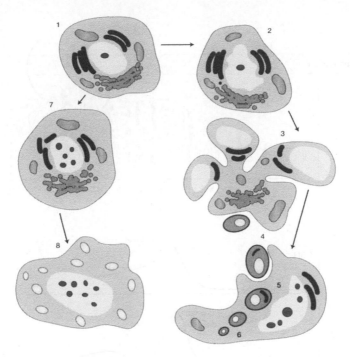

Figure 2.7 Schematic representation of ultrastructural changes in apoptosis (2–6) and necrosis (7–8).

2–6 Apoptosis
ATP consuming (endonucleases, other enzymes); no noxious conditions; single organellar groups are packaged into vesicles; typical morphological phenomena (blebbing, chromatin condensation and migration to the periphery, among others); macrophages clear out debris, but without local inflammation; examples: atresia, embryonal finger.

7–8 Necrosis
Process initiated by ATP deficiency; noxious conditions (ischemia, etc.); general swelling of the cell and disintegration of cell organelles; many special forms (colliquation, caseous degeneration, etc.); macrophages clear out debris with inflammatory consequences.
Adapted from reference 3

of the Graafian follicle and maximal pituitary LH release is approximately 24 hours. Ovulation follows on average 8–10 hours later. Midcycle physiological serum estradiol concentration is approximately 250 pg/ml.

An increase in serum LH concentration, which stimulates thecal cell androgen synthesis, occurs before the LH peak in the late follicular phase. This could possibly additionally increase the follicular epithelial cells' estradiol secretion. Luteinization of the follicular epithelial cells – evidenced by the onset of progesterone synthesis – begins prior to ovulation and is induced by rising LH and FSH levels. The LH peak is ended by the further increase in progesterone secretion (Figure 2.8).

17

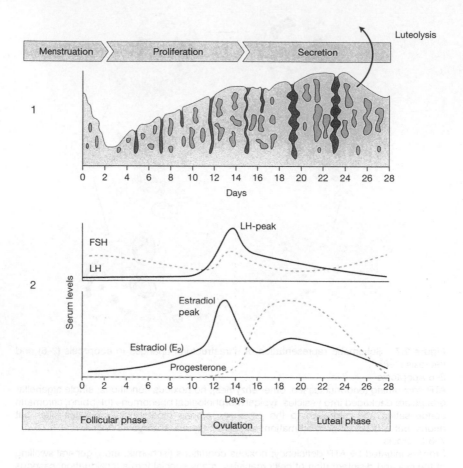

Figure 2.8 Morphological and endocrinological changes during the various phases of the cycle

CORPUS LUTEUM

The corpus luteum develops out of the ruptured follicle immediately following ovulation. The most important morphological characteristic of the corpus luteum is the pronounced vascularization of the previously avascular follicular epithelium (Figure 2.9). With its integration into the circulatory system and the expression of low-density lipoprotein (LDL) receptors, the follicular epithelial cells are able to take up cholesterol from the periphery and use it for progesterone biosynthesis. Serum progesterone values reach a peak of approximately 15 ng/ml at 6–8 days post-ovulation.

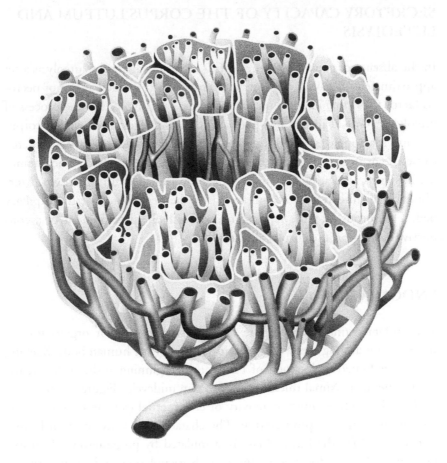

Figure 2.9 Vascularization of the corpus luteum shortly after ovulation: capillaries penetrate the individual lobes, which are separated from one another by fine connective tissue

CORPUS LUTEUM GRAVIDITATIS

In the event of fertilization, human chorionic gonadotropin (hCG) induces formation of the corpus luteum graviditatis. The hCG molecule is related to LH, having identical α-subunits but β-subunits with 31 additional amino acids. This additional peptide portion contains four additional carbohydrate chains.

The corpus luteum's main endocrine product is progesterone. Beside this, the corpus luteum is also capable of secreting limited amounts of estradiol.

SECRETORY CAPACITY OF THE CORPUS LUTEUM AND LUTEOLYSIS

In the absence of conception, the corpus luteum degrades by luteolysis after approximately 14 days. Cytokines and growth factors (such as tumor necrosis factor (TNF)-α) in addition to eicosanoids are involved in the process of luteolysis[6]. GnRH might also play a role in the degradation of the corpus luteum. Macrophages, which migrate into the corpus luteum, are considered to be the main source of the mediators involved in luteolysis. The chemotactic signals regulating this macrophage invasion remain unknown. Morphologically, luteolysis is accompanied by the degradation of the capillary bed. The corpus luteum's regression ends with the development of a connective tissue scar, the corpus albicans.

ENDOMETRIUM

The endometrium is one of the most important effector organs for sex steroids. It is among the fastest growing tissues of the human body. Starting with an endometrial thickness of 1 mm at the beginning of the cycle, the tissue reaches its maximal thickness of 7–8 mm midcycle (Figure 2.10).

Estradiol induces mitotic activity of endometrial cells, leading to a correspondingly massive proliferation. The characteristic secretory transformation required for the luteal phase is stimulated by progesterone. Transformation of the glandular epithelium, with vacuolation and an increase in glycogen storage and glandular secretion, takes place as early as the first week of the luteal phase. The conditions required for blastocyst implantation are thereby fulfilled. In the absence of fertilization, endometrium is sloughed off with menstruation.

The proliferative effect of estradiol on the endometrium is mediated by intracytoplasmic receptors. When the estradiol hormone receptor complex binds to DNA, the effects of this complex as a transcription factor cause transcription and translation of corresponding genes. As a result, proteins such as estrogen and progesterone receptors are synthesized. In addition, this cascade also causes various other growth factors to be synthesized, which stimulate endometrial proliferation by auto- and paracrine mechanisms. Thus, estradiol causes the induction of its own receptor, as well as the expression of progesterone receptors[7]. This sensitizes the endometrium to progesterone.

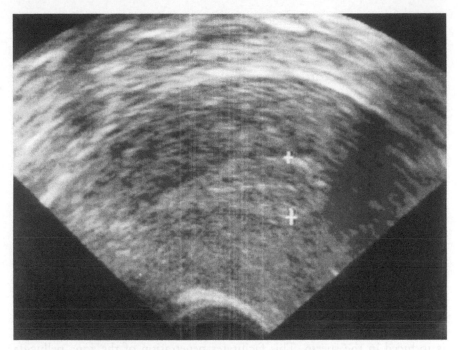

Figure 2.10 Ultrasound scan with longitudinal view of the uterus. Endometrial thickness is measured (+–+). Typical picture of the endometrium at midcycle

FERTILIZATION AND IMPLANTATION

Sperm transport

Sperm transport through the male genital tract is passive. It is not until passage through the epididymis that sperm attain their own mobility. After ejaculation, sperm transport is a combination of active and passive motility. The acidic vaginal environment (pH 3.5–5.5) is made more alkaline by seminal fluid. Sperm reach the cervix only a few minutes after ejaculation, and penetrate the cervical mucus at a rate of 2–3 mm per minute. In addition, pump-like uterine contractions passively transport sperm. This explains why motile sperm have been demonstrated in the Fallopian tubes only a few minutes after sexual intercourse.

The cervix also plays a storage role for sperm. Motile sperm are sequestered into cervical crypts and are gradually released for up to 3 days. Avital sperm are separated and subjected to phagocytosis in the cervix. Sperm can survive for up to 5 days in cervical crypts under optimal conditions. The ability of sperm to penetrate cervical mucus is cycle-dependent, and thereby hormone-dependent. Penetration of the mucus is not possible before the 9th day of the cycle and again 2–3 days after ovulation. Passage of sperm through the cavum uteri occurs relatively rapidly. Uterotubal transition is yet another barrier for sperm. Sperm transport in the Fallopian tube occurs in the opposite direction to egg cell transport and is regulated partially by active motility and partially by tubal contractions. Therefore, sperm also gain entry to the abdominal cavity through the Fallopian tubes. Sperm are generally demonstrable in the Douglas fluid a few hours after sexual intercourse.

Capacitation

Capacitation refers to the destabilization of the plasma cell membrane of the spermatozoon head (Figure 2.11). Sperm capacitate during their passage through the female genital tract. This occurs predominantly because of cholesterol withdrawal. Further, progesterone causes a massive calcium influx into the sperm, which changes the movement pattern. A hyperactive status is induced in the sperm. This facilitates penetration of the zona pellucida and is a preparation for the acrosome reaction. The acrosome reaction is physiologically triggered by the spermatozoon's contact with the zona pellucida. The outer acrosomal and plasma membranes fuse, with subsequent release of hyaluronidase and acrosin. Hyaluronidase and acrosin have lytic effects and facilitate the penetration of the zona pellucida.

Fertilization

The egg is captured by the fimbrial funnel of the Fallopian tube after ovulation and is transported through the Fallopian tubes toward the uterus by contractions.

The follicular epithelium of the cumulus oophorus surrounding the egg is separated during tubal transport. The zona pellucida remains, which is a glycoprotein layer 3–15 μm thick. As soon as the spermatozoon has undergone the acrosome reaction after contact with the zona pellucida, it enters the perivitelline space, fuses with the egg cell membrane, and is then incorporated (Figure 2.12). The egg releases subcortical granules during this process, which inactivate subsequent spermatozoa and make the zona pellucida impermeable to subsequent spermatozoa. This mechanism prevents multiple fertilization of the egg.

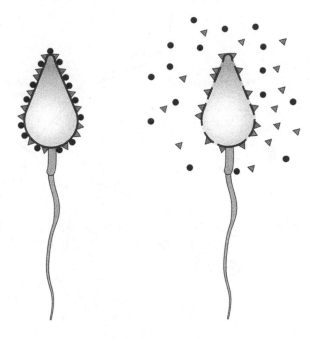

Figure 2.11 Schematic representation of the process of capacitation. The cell membrane is destabilized by cholesterol withdrawal

Binding of a spermatozoon to the zona pellucida is species specific, which is the reason why there are few animal species that can be crossed. Perhaps the most well-known interspecies cross is that between horse and donkey. The offspring of such a cross are sterile. Among felines, fertilization can be achieved by *in vitro* crossing of a lion and domestic cat, but the embryo dies after a few cleavage divisions. The creation of chimeras capable of reproduction is thereby prevented by these natural mechanisms.

Anatomically, fertilization most commonly takes place at the isthmo-ampullar transition of the Fallopian tube, where the first cleavage steps occur. In this early phase of development, the embryo is nourished only by pyruvate and lactate, both of which derive from the uterine environment. Differentiation of the blastomere occurs after the third cleavage step into the eight-cell stage. Transport of the embryo into the uterus occurs mostly during the late morula or early blastocyst stage. The embryo reaches the cavum uteri at 4 days post-conception at the earliest. In the blastocyst, an embryoblast surrounded by a trophoblastic cell corona is discernible (Figure 2.13).

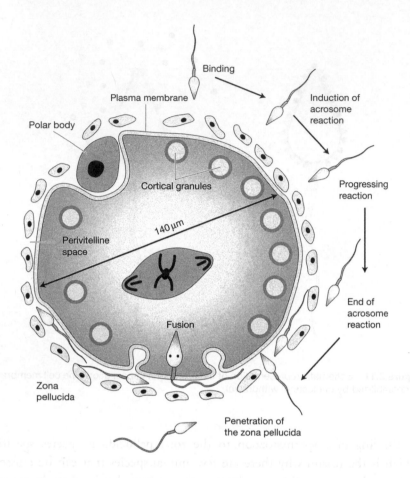

Figure 2.12 Schematic representation of the process of fertilization

The embryoblast finally separates from the zona pellucida in order to implant into the endometrium.

Time point of nidation

Implantation usually occurs on the 6th day post-conception (range 5.9–7.5 days). The syncytiotrophoblast and the cytotrophoblast can then be differentiated. The syncytiotrophoblast grows invasively into the endometrial stroma, the decidua. This leads to the erosion of blood vessels. The endometrium has wholly engulfed and closed over the implantation site on the 12th day post-conception, thereby completing the nidation process

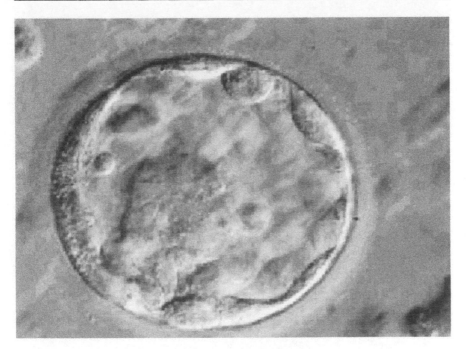

Figure 2.13   (See also Color Plate 1) The human blastocyst

(Figure 2.14). Trophoblast invasion into the endometrial stroma is specifically regulated; trophoblast invasion-limiting mechanisms are of special importance. Human uteroglobin apparently plays a key role. Uteroglobin exerts an anti-inflammatory effect on the nidation site, preventing neutrophil and monocyte infiltration into the nidation bed. However, it also binds to trophoblast cells to prevent an uncontrolled invasion[8].

Embryo–maternal dialogue

The human embryo starts its own metabolism at the eight-cell stage. It produces its own growth factors, interleukins and other cytokines which regulate the nidation process through para- and autocrine mechanisms. Maternal immune defense must be modulated in order to prevent the semi-allogenic embryo from being recognized as 'foreign' and rejected. The complementary system and leukemia inhibitory factor (LIF) are of special importance for the regulation of these complex immunological processes[9,10]. It is now known that the attachment of the embryo to the decidual surface is guided by local processes. Special proteins must be expressed and secreted

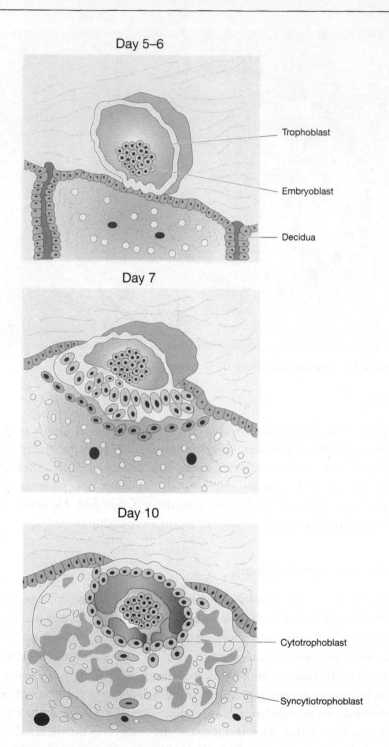

Figure 2.14 The process of implantation

into the extracellular matrix. Oncofetal fibronectin appears to play a particularly important role here.

The process of implantation and the aforementioned processes are genetically determined. Precise tuning of maternal and paternal gene activations is required. An exclusively paternal activation can lead to a uteroglobin coupling dysfunction, and thereby to unhindered trophoblast invasion. Furthermore, the embryonic chromosome number plays a decisive role. Aneuploid embryos can develop until the early morula stage, but perish soon afterwards. The aneuploidy rate increases with maternal age. This is one of the reasons for the age-dependent reduction in female fertility.

REFERENCES

1. De La Iglesia HO, Schwartz WJ. Timely ovulation: circadian regulation of the female hypothalamo–pituitary–gonadal axis. Endocrinology 2005; 147: 1148–53
2. Lanzone A, Fulghesu AM, Cucinelli F, et al. Evidence of a distinct derangement of opioid tone in hyperinsulinemic patients with PCOS. J Clin Endocrinol Metab 1995; 80: 3501–6
3. Keck C, Neulen J, Behre HM, Breckwoldt M. Endokrinologie Reproduktionsmedizin, Andrologie. Stuttgart: Thieme, 2002
4. Rolaki A, Drakakis P, Millingos S, et al. Novel trends in follicular development, atresia and corpus luteum regression: a role for apoptosis. Reprod Biomed Online 2005; 11: 93–103
5. Chun SY, Eisenhauer KM, Minami S, et al. Hormonal regulation of apoptosis in early antral follicles: follicle-stimulating hormone as a major survival factor. Endocrinology 1996; 137: 1447–56
6. Okuda K, Sakumoto R. Multiple roles of TNF super family members in corpus luteum function. Reprod Biol Endocrinol 2003; 1: 95
7. Katzenellenbogen BS. Mechanisms of action and cross-talk between estrogen receptor and progesterone receptor pathways. J Soc Gynecol Invest 2000; 7: 33–7
8. Beier HM. The discovery of uteroglobin and its significance for reproductive biology and endocrinology. Ann N Y Acad Sci 2000; 923: 9–24
9. Kimber SJ. Leukaemia inhibitory factor in implantation and uterine biology. Reproduction 2005; 130: 131–45
10. Nachtigall MJ, Kliman HJ, Feinberg RF, et al. The effect of leukemia inhibitory factor (LIF) on trophoblast differentiation: a potential role in human implantation. J Clin Endocrinol Metab 1996; 81: 801–6

3

Investigation of the infertile couple

HISTORY

Taking the medical history of the infertile couple in a personal interview should be the first step of every interaction between affected individuals and their treating physician. Besides building a personal relationship and establishing mutual trust and respect, the medical history is necessary to obtain critical information for planning the most relevant, useful, and cost-efficient diagnostic and therapeutic procedures.

Taking a medical history efficiently is an art, but some practical advice may be useful. The history-taking physician should be trained to adhere to a structured, reproducible and time-effective documentation of information. The interview should ideally incorporate both partners of the affected couple, be precise, documented in a reproducible written form, and performed within a given time frame. Patients should be asked beforehand to provide all related and medically relevant documents, in order to reduce common problems related to lay terminology and redundant diagnostic tests.

Table 3.1 suggests a checklist of items that may be specifically asked for during the interview of the infertile couple.

Some authors have suggested using a structured questionnaire containing all relevant questions. This approach has advantages such as standardization of information and time efficacy. On the other hand, studies have shown that self-reported information is less accurate compared with a personal interview. For example, Bergmann et al. compared the amount of information on personal disease history generated by personal interviews versus a self-administered questionnaire in 7481 participants[1]. They demonstrated that agreement between interview and questionnaire varied widely. Specifically, poor agreement was observed for less severe and more transient diseases, which were reported significantly more frequently in the personal

Table 3.1 Suggested checklist for taking a medical history of the infertile couple

Both partners

Age
Occupation, occupational hazards
Family history, e.g. hereditary diseases, cancer, thrombosis
Personal health problems
Current/past regular medications, substance abuse
Allergy
Previous surgery
Pregnancies, births

Woman

Age at menarche
Menstrual cycle details
Duration of infertility
Sexual activity and problems, e.g. dyspareunia
Hirsutism, acne, galactorrhea
Enlarged thyroid gland, tiredness

interview but not in the questionnaire. Based on this investigation and other related studies, it seems reasonable to recommend the use of structured medical history questionnaires only as a supplement to a structured personal interview.

MALE INFERTILITY

Infertility is defined as failure to conceive after 1 year of regular, unprotected intercourse. In 50–60% of the couples presenting with infertility a 'male factor' (or co-factor) can be identified. Thus, andrological knowledge is a condition *sine qua non* for medical doctors treating infertile couples. In many countries it is still a matter of debate who should investigate the infertile male, as there is no structured training in andrology available. In most countries the investigation is performed by reproductive medicine specialists, clinical andrologists or urologists.

The diagnostic management of the infertile male is not so different from the investigation in the female and comprises:

- History

- General examination

- Genital examination

- Hormone analysis

Specific for the male is the semen analysis, which is a key parameter of the investigation.

History

The information required concerns the duration of infertility, the frequency and effectiveness of coitus, pubertal development, any history of general disease or genitourinary infection or surgery. Furthermore, questions are posed concerning current medication, life-style factors and the reproductive outcome of previous partnerships.

General examination/genital examination

A thorough physical examination provides an overview of all organ systems and diseases which may be associated with hypogonadism and/or infertility. If androgen deficiency exists at the time of normal onset of puberty, eunuchoid tall stature results. The arm span exceeds the body length and the legs become longer than the trunk (Figure 3.1). Onset of androgen deficiency after puberty does not lead to a change of body proportions. Androgen deficiency as such does not directly cause an increase in subcutaneous fat tissue; however, fat distribution shows female characteristics.

Other symptoms of hypogonadism which can easily be detected are a straight frontal hairline, lacking or sparse beard growth (Figure 3.2) and a horizontal pubic hairline. In some cases gynecomastia can be found as a symptom of hypogonadism. However, gynecomastia has to be differentiated from lipomastia.

During genital examination the size, shape and consistency of the testes are evaluated. Extremely small but firm testes might indicate Klinefelter's syndrome, whereas soft testes of normal or decreased size might indicate a primary or secondary deterioration of spermatogenesis. Testicular volume is normally 12–30 ml per testis. Clinically this can be evaluated by palpation (Figure 3.3) using the Prader Orchidometer; application of ultrasound provides an objective measurement of testicular volume.

In addition to the evaluation of testes, palpation allows the diagnosis of aberrations in the epididymis, the pampiniform plexus and the deferent duct. A common finding is a varicocele, a distension of the venous

31

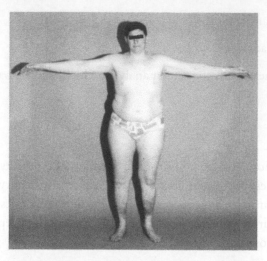

Figure 3.1 A 45-year-old patient with Klinefelter's syndrome. Arm span exceeds body length

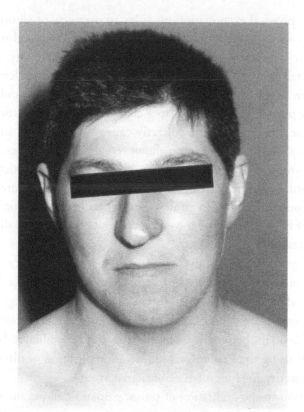

Figure 3.2 (See also Color Plate 2) A 45-year-old patient with Klinefelter's syndrome and characteristic straight frontal hairline and lacking beard growth

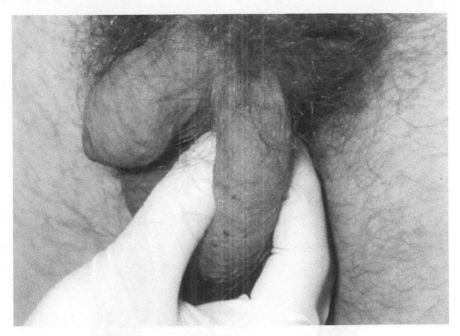

Figure 3.3   Palpation of the plexus pampiniformis

pampiniform plexus, usually appearing on the left side. Varicoceles are classified according to the following grades:

- Grade I can be palpated only during the Valsalva maneuver

- Grade II can be palpated without a Valsalva maneuver

- Grade III is a visible distension of the pampiniform plexus (Figure 3.4)

During examination of the penis, the location of the urethral orifice must be identified as dystopic localization, as seen in patients with epispadias or hypospadias, that might lead to fertility problems. Also, a phimosis or deviation of the penis during erections might negatively influence reproductive functions.

Hormone analysis

Whereas in the female, hormone analysis plays an essential role in the diagnostic algorithm, this is not the case for the male: the incidence of endocrine disorders as etiological factors for male infertility is extremely low and therefore only occasionally can causal treatment of male infertility be based on hormone analysis.

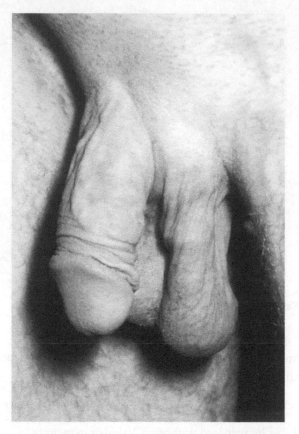

Figure 3.4   Varicocele III degree. Clearly visible through the scrotal skin

For basic diagnosis it is usually sufficient to determine testosterone, follicle stimulating hormone (FSH) and luteinizing hormone (LH) serum concentrations, as this provides information for specifying the cause of hypogonadism which is important for adequate therapy. High gonadotropin levels in combination with low testosterone levels indicate a testicular origin of hypogonadism (primary hypogonadism). Low gonadotropin levels point to a central cause (secondary hypogonadism). Only in special cases is an expansion of the spectrum of hormone measurements indicated: if the patient reveals clinical symptoms of hyperprolactinemia, hyper- or hypothyroidism or dysfunction of the adrenal gland, the respective analyses should be carried out. If, despite normal or even elevated testosterone levels, clinical symptoms of hypogonadism are detected, specific analysis of the testosterone receptor should be initiated. These analyses and particulary the interpretation of the results and the specific treatment should be performed by endocrinologists. They certainly do not belong to the basic repertoire of the reproductive medicine specialist.

Semen analysis

As indicated above, semen analysis is of key importance for evaluation of the infertile male. Different classification systems for the evaluation of semen and/or the semen–cervical mucus interaction have been developed, such as the World Health Organization (WHO) and the Tygerberg or 'strict' criteria. The most widely used classification system is probably that of the WHO, the latest version of which was published in 1999[2]. Although it is common knowledge today that semen analysis should be done under standardized conditions, it is important to realize that results of semen analysis can vary significantly even between different specialized centers. What does this mean for the clinical management of the infertile male? It means that one should not base the recommendation for a specific treatment on a single semen analysis. To be able to determine semen quality at least two or three analyses are needed.

The main parameters assessed during routine semen analysis are:

- Ejaculate volume

- Liquification time

- Sperm concentration

- Sperm motility

- Sperm morphology

- Presence of leukocytes in semen

Normal values for the above-mentioned parameters are available. However, it should be noted that, due to the subjective nature of the assessment, a huge variability for most of the parameters measured has to be taken into consideration.

Ejaculate volume can be measured either by collecting the specimen in graduated containers or by the use of a graduated pipette. Normal ejaculate volume is > 2 ml. If the volume is clearly below this threshold, then short abstinence time or malfunction of accessory glands or obstruction of their ducts might be the reason. More specific diagnostics are needed to reveal the origin of these conditions.

Normally semen liquefies within 30 minutes. If liquification time is significantly reduced or prolonged this might again indicate a malfunction of the accessory glands, such as prostate or seminal vesicles, and should be followed with specific tests.

Sperm concentration or sperm density is usually analyzed using specific counting chambers. A number of counting chambers are available, such as the hemocytometer, the Makler counting chamber, or the MicroCell chamber. Today in many laboratories computerized systems are available (see below).

The lower limit of sperm concentration as defined by WHO (1999)[2] is 20 million/ml. A sperm concentration lower than this is classified as oligozoospermia and some authors define grades of oligozoospermia according to the degree of reduction of sperm concentration (grade I–III). As already mentioned for semen volume, in cases of low sperm concentration the abstinence time should be verified, as a drastically shortened abstinence time might significantly reduce sperm concentration even in a male with otherwise normal spermatogenesis.

For analysis of sperm motility usually 200 sperm cells are evaluated and categorized according to their motility pattern graded as A–D. Owing to the subjective nature of this assessment a significant variability of results has to be taken into consideration and adequate quality control instruments have to be applied within the andrology laboratory to keep variability within an acceptable range. WHO defines 'normal motility' as at least 50% of sperm in grade A + B or 25% of sperm in grade A. If sperm motility falls below the above-mentioned thresholds the result is classified as asthenozoospermia.

Sperm morphology can be assessed not only by different classification systems (WHO, Tygerberg, etc.); but also within a classification system different staining methods are sometimes used. This certainly influences the results of the analysis, therefore sperm morphology is the parameter with the greatest variability among different centers.

In their manual WHO defined 30% 'normal sperm' as the lower threshold. However, nowadays this threshold is certainly questionable and discussions are ongoing to clarify whether a different 'normal range' needs to be defined.

Besides or instead of the WHO classification many laboratories use the Tygerberg (Kruger) criteria for assessing sperm morphology[3]. With this classification system normal morphology of 15% or greater would be considered as a normal result.

Leukocytes in semen are usually detected by the peroxidase staining method, which provides a cheap and simple way of quantification. However, with this method no differentiation of leukocyte subtypes is possible. For routine use differentiation is not necessary, as the peroxidase method is sufficient to differentiate between a significantly elevated concentration of leukocytes, which requires further diagnostic and therapeutic follow-up, and a normal range of leukocytes (Figure 3.5).

Beyond the sperm parameters mentioned above a variety of other investigations can be performed which give a more detailed characterization of the semen quality, such as biochemical analyses or electron microscopic evaluations. However, with the exception of determination of marker substances in order to diagnose seminal tract obstruction, these specific methods usually have no influence on the therapeutic options for the patient, and therefore these diagnostic tests will not be discussed here. Similarly, some laboratories apply computerized assessment of semen analysis (CASA) which is an interesting tool for research purposes but has not yet replaced the typical 'manual' semen analysis outlined above. Therefore, discussion of different CASA technologies available will be left to the specific literature.

Antisperm antibodies have received a great deal of attention in previous years and different systems were developed to detect antisperm antibodies in body fluids and in the female genital tract. In spite of extensive research and several studies exploring strategies to reduce the level of antisperm antibodies there has never been sufficient evidence that this resulted in an improved reproductive outcome. Therefore, today, routine testing of antisperm antibodies and/or treatment of this condition can be seen as obsolete.

Similarly to the measurement of antisperm antibodies in previous years, multiple 'sperm function tests' were applied such as the hypo-osmotic swelling test, the eosin test, the zona-binding test, etc. In the era of *in vitro* fertilization (IVF) and intracytoplasmic sperm injection (ICSI) most of these functional tests have completely lost their relevance, as a significant correlation between test results and outcome of these procedures could not be demonstrated.

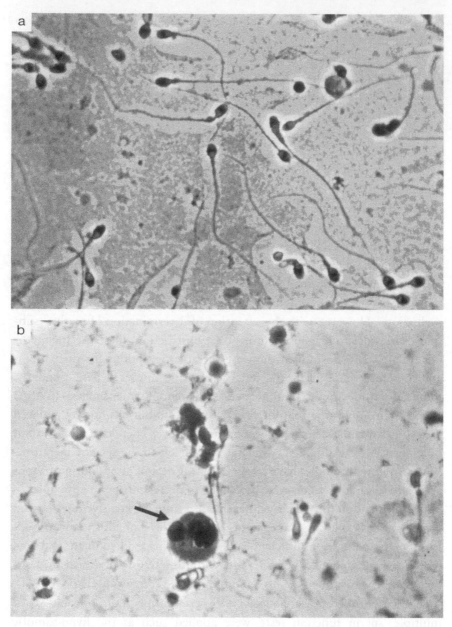

Figure 3.5 (See also Color Plate 3) (a) Normal sperm morphology; (b) detection of a leukocyte by peroxidase staining;

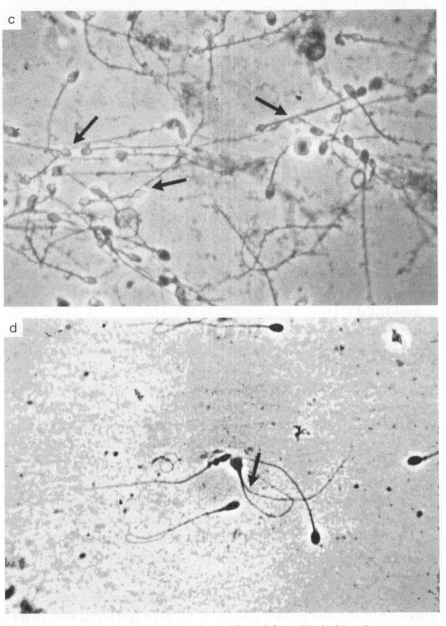

Figure 3.5 *Continued* (c) acrosome defects; (d) tail defect with double tail

Therapeutic options in male infertility

As in other medical fields, the treatment of male infertility should be based on diagnosis of the underlying disease. There are several situations where causal treatment of male infertility can be applied, e.g. in cases of seminal tract infections or in the (although rare) cases of hypogonadotropic gonadism, etc. However, no matter what type of diagnostic algorithm is applied, approximately 40% of infertile male patients will be classified as 'idiopathic infertile' which means that the etiology of their infertility remains unclear and therefore obviously a causal treatment is not available.

In the past a variety of different conservative treatments have been applied to idiopathic male infertility; however, none of these treatments could demonstrate a significant improvement of patients' fertility.

Pulsatile gonadotropin releasing hormone (GnRH) treatment was suggested in patients with oligoasthenoteratozoospermia and elevated FSH levels, but an improvement in semen parameters and/or pregnancy rates has not been demonstrated[4].

Androgens were applied, as it was believed that in men with idiopathic infertility following treatment with testosterone spermatogenic activity would be increased, resulting in elevated sperm concentration compared with pretreatment values (so-called rebound effect). This concept, however, could never be confirmed and was therefore abandoned.

Antiestrogens and *aromatase inhibitors* such as clomiphene or tamoxifen have been tried in the treatment of idiopathic male infertility. The inefficacy of all these compounds has been shown in several controlled prospective trials[5].

Kallikrein was used on a large scale for the treatment of idiopathic infertility, although a clear pathophysiological or pharmacological concept was missing. At the beginning of the 1990s two randomized placebo-controlled prospective studies[6,7] came to the conclusion that kallikrein had no beneficial effect on male idiopathic infertility.

Pentoxyphyllin belongs to the family of methylxanthines and leads to relaxation of vascular smooth muscles. It has been speculated that, in men with idiopathic infertility, testicular circulation might be disturbed and would be improved by pentoxyphyllin. However, there is no evidence for circulatory disturbances in idiopathic infertility nor is there proof of any clear therapeutic effect of pentoxyphyllin.

In almost all fields of medicine oxidative damage of proteins and nucleic acids is being discussed as a major contributing factor in aging/

degenerative diseases. Furthermore, in the field of fertility disorders, the use of *antioxidative agents* has been considered. Although an effect could be shown on specific sperm parameters, there is no evidence to date that the use of antioxidants improves sperm function overall or patients' fertility potential.

EXAMINATION OF THE FEMALE INFERTILITY PATIENT

A thorough physical examination of the female infertility patient has been proposed by some authors to be included in the routine diagnostic work-up. On the other hand, body structure, height, weight (body mass index; BMI), distribution of hair growth, galactorrhea and acne can be assessed by direct questioning and inspection during the gynecological examination, making a whole-body physical examination unnecessary.

Obesity is associated with reduced fertility and fecundity[8]. Therefore, an evaluation and documentation of the BMI should be routine. The Institute of Medicine, National Academy of Sciences, defines obesity as a BMI of > 29, a BMI between 19.8 and 26 as normal, a BMI between 26 and 29 as high, and a BMI of < 19.8 as low[9] (Figure 3.6).

Obesity is associated with various specific pathologies relevant to the gynecological endocrinologist, among them oligomenorrhea, amenorrhea, anovulation, insulin resistance and polycystic ovary syndrome (PCOS) (Figure 3.7). Furthermore, a low BMI is associated with an increased risk of ovarian dysfunction or failure[10]. Therefore, the BMI can give important clues to a number of possible causes of infertility. The routine evaluation and documentation of the BMI is also important to track changes of the BMI used as a therapeutic intervention. For example, in obese women with clomiphene-resistant anovulation, a reduction of the BMI significantly increases the rate of ovulation, improves insulin sensitivity and reduces serum levels of androgens[11,12].

A gynecological examination including inspection, bimanual palpation and transvaginal ultrasonography should be part of the routine diagnostic work-up of the infertility patient. The goal of the gynecological examination in this context is to rule out anatomical anomalies and local pathologies, precluding or requiring further treatment such as local infections, adnexal masses, cervical cancer/pathology and congenital anomalies, e.g. hymenal

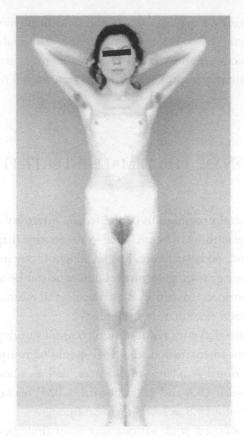

Figure 3.6   An 18-year-old patient with anorexia nervosa and amenorrhea

atresia, adrenogenital syndrome (AGS), or Mayer–Rokitansky–Kuester–Hauser syndrome (Figure 3.8).

Basal body temperature chart

The basal body temperature chart (BBTC) has been traditionally used to test whether or not ovulation has occurred and to estimate the time of ovulation. This diagnostic test is based on the fact that the secretion of progesterone by the corpus luteum increases the body temperature by approximately 0.5°C. The biochemical mechanism of sex steroid-dependence of body temperature is not clear. It has been proposed that γ-aminobutyric acid (GABA)-mediated transmission in the medial preoptic area (MPOA) of the hypothalamus may be the critical factor in this respect[13]. Temperature can be

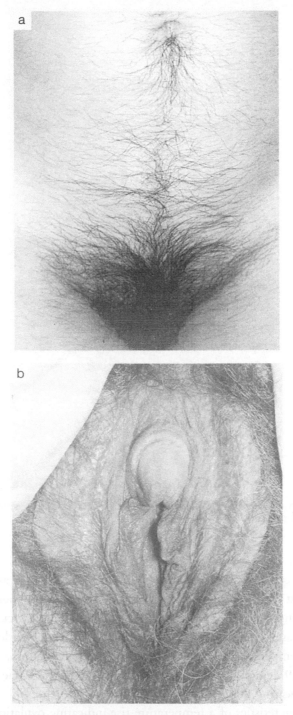

Figure 3.7   A 31-year-old patient with PCOS. Hirsutism (a) and enlargement of the clitoris (b) as symptoms of hyperandrogenism

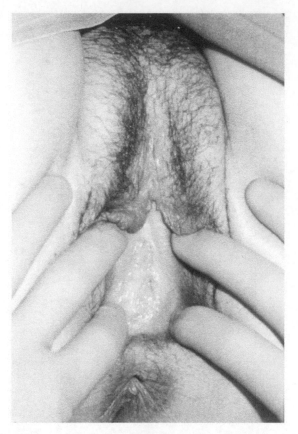

Figure 3.8 A 34-year-old patient with Rokitansky–Küster–Mayer syndrome. Typical aspect of the introitus

measured rectally, orally, vaginally, or in the axil, as long as the site of measurement is not changed during a given cycle. Measurements are taken every morning. The BBTC is expected to depict a biphasic curve with the follicular phase at the lower and the luteal phase at the higher level. The day before the temperature rise is considered the day of ovulation.

Figure 3.9 demonstrates a BBTC with a sustained midcycle temperature increase indicating that ovulation has occurred.

The characteristics of a temperature rise indicating ovulation have been defined variously. For example, one definition requires the temperature

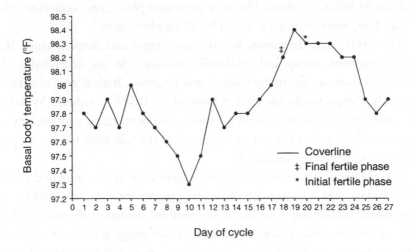

Figure 3.9 Basal body temperature chart. Adapted from reference 14, with permission from Elsevier

reading to be at least 0.2°C higher during three continuous days compared with the 6 days before. Another definition asks for a temperature rise of 0.4–0.6°C on one day with a following sustained temperature elevation. In addition, it is possible to combine the female and male temperatures in order to minimize the influence of non-specific, exogenous influences on the body temperature, which are presumably shared by the couple. This interpretation technique uses the difference between the couple's temperature readings, called the 'Gap' technique. Lang Dunlop *et al.* compared the two BBTC interpretation techniques, i.e. the 'Gap' (female and male) and the 'Coverline' (female) techniques in a series of 38 cycles[14]. In this study, there was no difference between the two techniques regarding the identification of the postovulatory fertile period (39% vs. 30% of cycles, respectively). In contrast, the postovulatory infertile phase, defined as beginning on the third day after the presumed day of ovulation, was identified within +1 day of that of LH testing in 13/33 (39%) and 4/33 (12%) cycles, respectively ($p < 0.001$). The 'Gap' and 'Coverline' techniques overestimated the fertile period by 1 and 4 days, respectively ($p = 0.0002$). Based on this small study, the 'Gap' technique appears to be more accurate in identifying the postovulatory infertile phase, but not the preovulatory fertile period.

The interpretation of a BBTC has its difficulties, even for experts. In a study of 98 BBTCs evaluated by six experienced physicians, only nine (9%) of the charts were correctly assessed by all six physicians[15].

The BBTC as a diagnostic test has advantages and disadvantages. It is easy to perform, cheap and minimally invasive. On the other hand, the BBTC is a nuisance for many women and requires a high degree of compliance. Most importantly, the clinical value of the BBTC is reduced by its low sensitivity as a diagnostic tool for assessing the occurrence and the time of ovulation. This makes the test unacceptable as the sole basis for further procedures, e.g. ovarian stimulation.

In a series of 101 infertile women, Guermandi et al. compared BBTC with urinary LH testing, luteal serum progesterone measurements and transvaginal ultrasonography as the standard for ovulation detection[16]. Urinary LH testing and a single midluteal serum progesterone measurement were superior to the BBTC. Specifically, the urinary LH surge preceded follicular rupture in 97/97 cases, and serum progesterone showed ovulatory values (≥ 6 ng/ml) in 90/97 cases. In 11/101 women basal body temperature was not assessable. The basal body temperature showed a wide interindividual variability and the BBTC as a diagnostic tool for ovulation detection had a sensitivity of 0.77 and a specificity of 0.33. In a recent study using urinary LH measurement as standard, the BBTC identified the postovulatory fertile phase within ±1 day of that identified by LH testing in only 10/33 (30%) cycles[14].

These data indicate that the BBTC is of limited value for predicting ovulation because of its low sensitivity and wide variability, i.e. ovulation occurs between 6 days before and 4 days after the basal body temperature nadir. It has to be acknowledged, however, that the BBTC is useful, although with low specificity, for the confirmation of ovulation.

Owing to its shortcomings as a diagnostic test, the BBTC is not routinely used in the diagnostic work-up of the infertility patient. Today, the BBTC has been replaced by urinary LH testing and/or serum LH and progesterone measurements.

It has to be noted, however, that occasionally infertile patients may present to the physician with – sometimes meticulously designed – BBTCs. For the sake of clarity and intellectual correctness, these patients should be correctly instructed about the diagnostic value of this test. On the other hand, patients expect physicians to appreciate their own efforts and contributions to improve their condition. Therefore, the treating physician should be able and willing to interpret BBTCs, if they are available. For this reason, every physician involved in infertility treatment should be knowledgeable about the BBTC, even though it is not used in daily clinical practice.

The BBTC is also used by some women as a form of contraception. In this regard, the BBTC is also of limited value. For example, in a study of 142 women, contraception by BBTC had a high pregnancy/failure rate of 25% during a 12-month period compared with 0% with oral contraception (OC) and 2% with an intrauterine device (IUD)[17].

Hormone diagnostics

In most institutions, a comprehensive panel of hormone tests is assessed in order to identify the most common pathologies associated with infertility. In this respect, both the prevalence of the pathology defined by or indicated by a specific hormone test and the costs of a testing panel should be considered. For example, the most common causes of ovulatory dysfunction are: (1) PCOS (approximately 70% of cases of ovulatory dysfunction)[18]; (2) hyperprolactinemia (approximately 10% of cases); (3) hypothalamic amenorrhea, also known as hypogonadotropic hypogonadism (approximately 10% of cases); and (4) premature ovarian failure, also known as hypergonadotropic hypoestrogenic anovulation (approximately 10% of cases)[19].

In most institutions, a set of hormone tests is routinely performed in all patients with a diagnosis of primary or secondary sterility, defined as regular intercourse with or without a history of a previous pregnancy, respectively. It has never been proven, however, that the assessment of a specific set of hormones is necessary to achieve a high pregnancy rate or to reduce the time to pregnancy. Therefore, an evidence-based recommendation as to the composition of such an initial hormone panel cannot be given.

The specific composition of a hormone test panel must be defined by every institution, because questions of financial and technical resources, academic interest as well as local clinical practice vary widely and strongly influence the choice of specific hormone tests.

As with any diagnostic test, the assessment of a specific hormone should ideally provide an answer to a specific question. The aim of the initial diagnostic work-up of an infertility patient is to decide which treatment, if any, is appropriate in order to achieve a reasonable chance of pregnancy. It therefore seems appropriate to list the questions any panel of hormone tests should be able to answer.

Does the patient have PCOS and/or hyperandrogenemia?

According to an international consensus published in 2004[20], the diagnosis of PCOS is established by a combination of at least two of the following three items:

- Oligo-ovulation or anovulation (usually manifested as oligomenorrhea or amenorrhea)

- Elevated levels of circulating androgens (hyperandrogenemia) or clinical manifestations of androgen excess (hyperandrogenism)

- Polycystic ovaries as defined by ultrasonography

As to serum hormone testing, one part of the diagnosis of PCOS is based on the evaluation of serum testosterone (TES). Measurement of androstenedione is performed by many groups; however, it is not mentioned in the Rotterdam consensus. In women, 50%, 25% and 25% of serum TES is produced by the peripheral conversion of androstenedione to TES, ovarian production, and production in the adrenal cortex, respectively. One per cent of TES is found in the form of free TES, whereas 30–40% of TES is bound to albumin and 50–70% of TES is bound to sex hormone binding protein (SHBG).

When interpreting androgen measurements, it should be taken into account that commercial kits are not always reliable. Furthermore, it should be noted that age, BMI and smoking habits may have an effect on serum androgen levels.

Controversy exists regarding the necessity of the measurement of free TES and bioavailable TES. Free TES can be assessed by equilibrium analysis, but this technique is expensive. Thus, an indirect measurement of free TES, namely the free TES index (fTi), can be used according to the following formula:

$$fTi = 100 \times \frac{TES \, (nmol/l)}{SHBG \, (nmol/l)}$$

The fTi has been demonstrated to have a high correlation with free TES[21]. In summary, serum evaluation of TES and androstenedione in combination with transvaginal sonography, clinical assessment of symptoms of hyperandrogenemia, menstrual history and ovulation assessment are necessary to establish/rule out a diagnosis of PCOS and should therefore be part of the initial diagnostic work-up of a woman with infertility.

Table 3.2 demonstrates the reference values for serum TES, free TES and fTi.

Does the patient have hypogonadotropic hypogonadism?

Hypothalamic–pituitary failure or WHO group I ovarian failure is characterized by low serum concentrations of gonadotropins. Subsequently, no follicle development and ovarian steroidogenesis occurs. WHO group I ovarian failure can be diagnosed by measurement of serum LH and FSH. Table 3.3 demonstrates the reference values for LH and FSH. Overall, WHO group I ovarian insufficiency is a rare condition.

Does the patient have hyperprolactinemia and/or non-classical congenital adrenal hyperplasia?

A single measurement of serum 17-hydroxyprogesterone is usually sufficient to rule out non-classical congenital adrenal hyperplasia due to deficiency of 21-hydroxylase. It is important to measure the 17-hydroxyprogesterone level in a blood sample taken in the early morning, when endogenous corticotropin levels peak. As an alternative test, 17-hydroxyprogesterone can be measured in response to a single dose of exogenously administered corticotropin.

A single measurement of serum prolactin is usually sufficient to rule out hyperprolactinemia if the blood sample is taken under standardized conditions. Table 3.4 shows the reference values for serum prolactin.

Table 3.2 Reference values for serum testosterone (TES), free TES and the free TES index (fTi) in women	
	Value
TES	
Median age 37 (range 15–75) years	0.14–0.76 µg/l; 0.5–2.6 nmol/l
Free TES	
Reproductive phase	1–6 ng/l; 3.5–21 pmol/l
fTi	
Whole cycle	0.8–10
Midcycle	1.3–17

Table 3.3 Reference values for serum luteinizing hormone (LH) and follicle stimulating hormone (FSH) in women

	FSH (IU/l)	LH (IU/l)
Follicular phase	2.5–10.2	1.9–12.5
Periovulation	3.4–33.4	8.7–76.3
Luteal phase	1.5–9.1	0.5–16.9
Oral contraceptive use	<4.9	0.7–5.6
Pregnancy	<0.3	<1.5
Postmenopause	23–116.3	15.9–54

Table 3.4 Reference values of serum prolactin in women

Age	µg/l	mIU/l
4–11 years	2.6–21.0	62–504
12–13 years	2.5–16.9	60–406
14–18 years	4.2–39.0	101–936
Adults	3.8–23.2	91–557

Prolactin appears in several forms: 80–90% of prolactin is found in the form of 'little' prolactin. 'Little' prolactin has a molecular weight of 23 kDa and has the highest biological activity of all prolactin forms. Larger variants are generated by dimerization or building of a complex with other proteins. These forms of prolactin are called 'big' prolactin or 'bigbig' prolactin with a molecular weight of 150–170 kDa[22]. These larger prolactin variants are characterized by low biological activity. Prolactin variants can be identified by gel chromatography.

Clinically, hyperprolactinemia caused by large prolactin variants may lead to diagnostic discrepancies owing to the failure to detect 'big' prolactin. Subsequently, clinical symptoms of hyperprolactinemia can be associated with laboratory findings consistent with normoprolactinemia. On the other hand, clinically irrelevant laboratory findings of hyperprolactinemia due to increased concentrations of large prolactin variants can lead to unnecessary diagnostic and therapeutic interventions. Therefore, every laboratory involved in prolactin testing is required to use gel chromatography or polyethylene glycol (PEG) precipitation to differentiate between prolactin and prolactin variants[23]. When interpreting these laboratory findings, it has to be kept in mind that large prolactin variants have a low biological activity and cases of hyperprolactinemia with a proportion of 50% of large prolactin variants is mostly clinically irrelevant. In any case, the laboratory findings have to be interpreted in conjunction with the clinical symptoms.

Elevated serum concentrations of prolactin are found during pregnancy and lactation. If these conditions are ruled out, the likelihood of a prolactinoma is significantly increased with values of > 50 µg/l and relatively certain with values between 200 and 500 µg/l[24]. Rare prolactin concentrations of > 1000 µg/l are indicative of an invasive prolactinoma.

Alternatively, increased serum concentrations of prolactin with values up to 100 µg/l and above may be caused by drug use, e.g. antidepressants, neuroleptics, estradiol, antihypertensives, dopamine antagonists and opioids.

Hypothyroidism with elevated thyroid stimulating hormone (TSH) serum concentrations up to 40–50 µg/l may also lead to hyperprolactinemia by stimulation of pituitary prolactin secretion. Hyperandrogenemia and chronic stress have also been described to be associated with mild hyperprolactinemia[25,26].

Is the patient in a postmenopausal state?

By evaluating serum levels of estradiol and FSH, a pre- or postmenopausal state can be diagnosed. Hypoestrogenism and high concentrations of FSH in addition to amenorrhea constitute a diagnosis of WHO group III ovarian failure. Notwithstanding variations between laboratories, an estradiol concentration of < 20 pg/ml and an FSH concentration of > 25 IU/l can be considered supportive of this diagnosis. Of note, FSH concentrations between 3 and 30 IU/l are found around the time of ovulation. In the perimenopausal phase the first clinical feature of ovarian failure is usually a shortening of the follicular phase, which is currently explained by a sharp increase in serum FSH concentration during the luteal transition. In this situation, FSH serum concentrations at day 3 are usually within the normal range and an increased value of serum estradiol hints at the shortened follicular phase.

In case of a hormone constellation consistent with a postmenopausal state, the next step is to differentiate between natural menopause in women > 40 years of age, premature ovarian failure (POF) with an array of possible causes ranging from iatrogenic ovarian damage to steroidogenic autoimmune oophoritis, myasthenia gravis-related FSH receptor autoantibodies, or idiopathic POF[27].

Ultrasound

Usually the ultrasound evaluation starts with the assessment of the uterus. It should be visualized in its longest longitudinal plane. Thus, the maximal length from the cervix to the fundus and the length of the uterine cavity can be determined; this could be of importance when performing cervical catheterization prior to embryo transfer or intrauterine insemination.

Uterine malformations that have not been detected by palpation can easily be diagnosed by ultrasound. Aberrations from the normal shape of the organ due to the presence of fibromas or septations can be classified. If fibromas are detected, the size, localization and structure should be documented. Some fibromas could severely impair reproductive function, e.g. if they obstruct the Fallopian tube. Submucous fibromas could severely impair implantation conditions, depending on the size and localization (Figure 3.10).

Evaluation of the endometrial structure is crucial. Close to midcycle the endometrium normally shows a three-layer appearance with a distinct

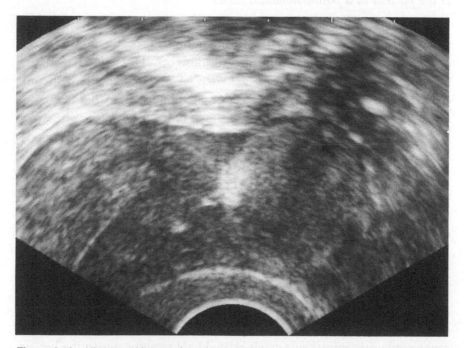

Figure 3.10 Ultrasound image of a subserous fibroma in the fundus uteri

'middle echo'. At this time the endometrium has a thickness of at least 8 mm. Endometrial thickness significantly below this level might indicate suboptimal implantation conditions and warrants further investigation. After ovulation, endometrial thickness decreases and the structure appears more dense.

For investigation of the endometrium it is crucial to choose the cycle period correctly: endometrial thickness should be evaluated at midcycle (Figure 3.11). Polyps or submucous fibromas can more easily be diagnosed directly after menses. Ultrasound investigations should therefore be scheduled accordingly.

Fallopian tubes

Normally the Fallopian tubes are not visible at ultrasound examination; they are only visible if distended (due to hydrosalpinx/pyosalpinx). The Fallopian tubes can be evaluated by methods using contrast media. This will be discussed below.

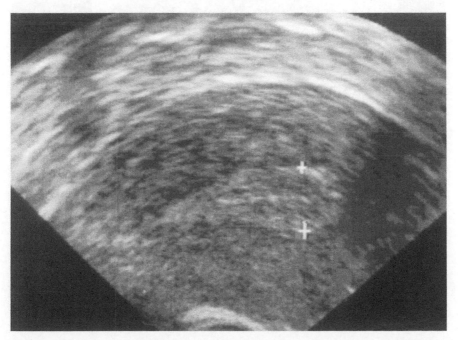

Figure 3.11 Ultrasound image of the typical three-layer appearance of the endometrium at midcycle

Ovaries

Ovarian size can be evaluated objectively by ultrasound. It clearly depends on female age. For women of reproductive age ovarian size is 4–5 cm in diameter and decreases progressively with age. In postmenopausal women sometimes the ovaries can hardly be detected due to a diameter below 1–2 cm. For clinical purposes it is usually sufficient to determine ovarian volume by measuring two perpendicular planes; however, most ultrasound machines provide programs to calculate the volume automatically.

Besides the size of the ovaries, ultrasound is used to detect ovarian cysts or aberrations of follicular development. As for the endometrium, it is important to interpret the results on the basis of the cycle phase in which the examination has been performed: in the early follicular phase usually a number of antral follicles (6–10) can be detected. During the menstrual cycle follicular development can be monitored. At the time of ovulation the leading

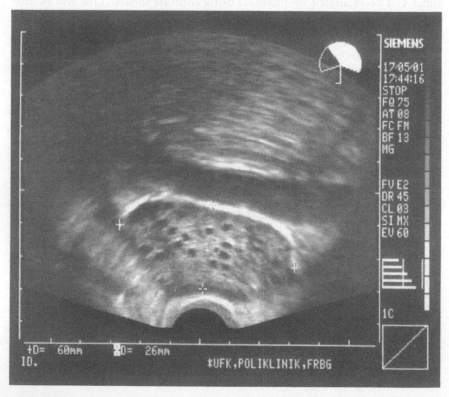

Figure 3.12　Ultrasound image of a polycystic ovary. Significant enlargement of the ovary with a diameter of 26 × 60 mm

follicle (in an unstimulated cycle) reaches a diameter of 22–25 mm whereas the other follicles remain clearly below this size. This picture is completely different in stimulated cycles and we will discuss this below.

Polycystic ovaries are a relatively common finding (Figure 3.12). It has been shown that polycystic ovaries can be found in 26% of women with amenorrhea, 87% with oligomenorrhea and 92% with hirsutism. In very young women shortly after puberty polycystic ovaries are even more common, even without the above-mentioned symptoms.

In the 'classical case' of PCOS multiple follicular cysts and increased stroma are found in ovaries that are usually, but not always, enlarged. This finding has a significant impact on future treatment strategies: in order to establish the diagnosis of PCOS the patient has to be examined carefully for symptoms of hyperandrogenism, androgen measurements must to be performed and a detailed menstrual cycle history must be taken. If the patient is diagnosed with PCOS various treatment options need to be discussed (see below).

Ovarian cysts are a common ultrasound finding. Especially in women who do not use oral contraceptives, ovarian cysts might appear spontaneously and they might also disappear spontaneously without any intervention. Ovarian cysts can be classified according to their nature:

- Corpus luteum cysts

- Functional cysts

- Multilocular cysts

Corpus luteum cysts result from blood influx into the follicular cavity after ovulation (Figure 3.13). These cysts can present with a bizarre appearance and they can occasionally reach a diameter of more than 10 cm. Corpus luteum cysts disappear spontaneously after menstruation.

Functional cysts derive from persistent follicles. They are usually unilocular. Functional cysts do not produce steroids; however, they can increase in size on gonadotropin treatment. Usually expectant management is adequate as these cysts disappear after 2–3 months. Only if they persist or exceed a certain size (> 4–5 cm) should surgical intervention be discussed. If functional cysts are detected immediately prior to ovarian stimulation, treatment should be delayed until the next cycle in order to wait for the cyst to disappear.

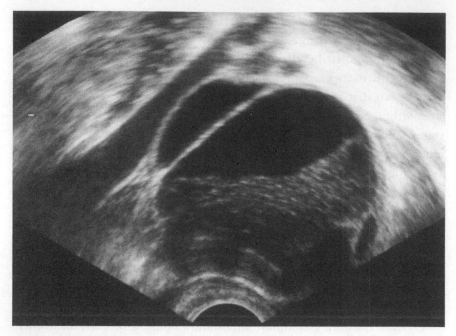

Figure 3.13 Ultrasound image of a corpus luteum cyst

If multilocular cysts are found, the differential diagnosis comprises ovarian endometriosis with septated cysts, dermoids or a hydrosalpinx.

If at ultrasound examination an adnexal mass of undefined nature is diagnosed, further diagnostic procedures are mandatory. Although in young women malign processes are extremely rare, in case of doubt the diagnosis has to be established via laparoscopy or open surgery.

Assessment of Fallopian tubes at conventional ultrasound examination

During normal ultrasound assessment the Fallopian tubes are not visible. However, when pathologically filled with fluid (hydrosalpinx) (Figure 3.14) or pus (pyosalpinx) the structures of the tubes can be detected. Hydrosalpinges are associated with an impairment of reproductive function. Therefore, if the hydrosalpinx persists over a longer period of time, it has to be decided whether an intervention is indicated. It is still a matter of debate whether hydrosalpinges should be removed initially or whether a distal salpingostomy, to allow peritoneal drainage of intratubal fluid, should be performed.

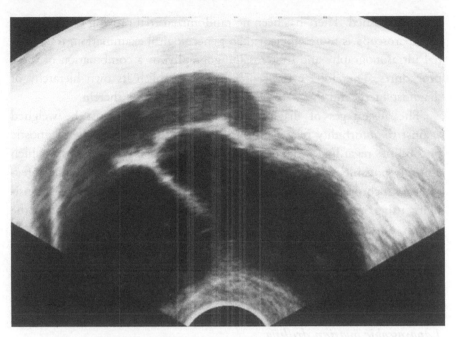

Figure 3.14 Ultrasound image of a hydrosalpinx in a 32-year-old patient with chronic pelvic infection (*Chlamydia* infection)

Assessment of Fallopian tube patency will be discussed below.

Laparoscopy

Today, laparoscopy is an integral part of diagnosis and therapy of infertility patients. Reproductive surgery has been established as a *de facto* subspecialization of gynecological endocrinology in many industrialized countries. A high-standard minimally invasive surgery unit should be part of every modern infertility treatment center. Specifically, the following procedures should be performed routinely and with an adequate frequency to allow for a specialized and quality-assured performance: diagnostic laparoscopy, laparoscopic myomectomy, ovarian drilling, tubal patency assessment, treatment of intra-abdominal adhesions, resection of endometriotic lesions and hysteroscopy.

Diagnostic laparoscopy

The value of diagnostic laparoscopy as a routine diagnostic method for infertility patients without clinically established or suspected pathology has not been established. There has been no randomized trial proving that diagnostic laparoscopy is more efficient than gynecological examination, transvaginal ultrasonography and hysterosalpingography, or a combination of these procedures. Therefore, every center has to establish its own hierarchy of diagnostic tests and the place of diagnostic laparoscopy therein.

The advantages of diagnostic laparoscopy, which must be weighed against the morbidity related to this surgical procedure, are the diagnostic possibilities regarding intra-abdominal adhesions and endometriosis, which are only possible with this procedure. In addition, intra-abdominal infections, e.g. chronic *Chlamydia* infection, are diagnosed with a higher sensitivity using intra-abdominal samples[28]. Moreover, laparoscopy offers the option of simultaneous diagnosis and treatment if such a pathology is present.

In our institution, we follow the current recommendations of experts in the field advocating the routine use of diagnostic laparoscopy if an intra-abdominal pathology is suspected[25].

Laparoscopic ovarian drilling

Laparoscopic ovarian drilling (LOD) is a surgical option to re-establish ovulation, which is used alone or in combination with medical ovarian stimulation[30]. Of note, surgical treatment of the ovary was the first treatment option for women described as having the Stein–Leventhal syndrome. From the 1930s until the introduction of laparoscopy, a partial resection of one-third of the ovaries, termed 'wedge resection' was the only available method besides weight reduction to treat affected women. 'Wedge resection' has a success rate of approximately 50%. Medical alternatives of ovarian stimulation, i.e. clomiphene and gonadotropins, as well as the high morbidity of 'wedge resection' regarding intra-abdominal adhesions in the order of 50–70% have led to the abandonment of this method[30].

LOD by diathermy or laser uses the same principles as 'wedge resection' and has been established as a standard method of treating women with clomiphene-resistant anovulation. LOD destroys androgen-producing ovarian theca cells, reduces serum androgen concentrations by 40%, reduces ovarian volume after an initial increase, reduces serum LH and increases serum FSH[31–33]. Some have claimed that LOD has a high long-term success rate of up to 70% after 10 years[34]. This is another advantage of LOD versus medical ovarian stimulation.

The role of this treatment option in the hierarchy of treatment options, however, is controversial. LOD is less expensive and has a lower risk of multiple pregnancies compared to medical treatment. Farquhar[35] evaluated the economics of both treatments. The total cost of treatment in this analysis was E 4664 for the ovarian drilling group and E 5418 for the gonadotropin group. Without the cost of monitoring and the diagnostic laparoscopy then the difference was E 2110 in favor of ovarian drilling. It was estimated that the cost per term pregnancy would be E 14 489 for gonadotropin and E 11 301 for ovarian drilling (22% lower). Advantages of the surgical method are a lower risk of multiple pregnancy and the positive long-term effect of LOD on ovulatory capacity. On the other hand, LOD carries a small, but significant, risk of operative morbidity and intra-abdominal adhesions of around 20–40%. In addition, another medical option of ovulation induction, namely metformin, has been reported to reduce the rates of miscarriage by 30%[36]. This effect is not found after LOD.

Many uncontrolled observational studies have claimed that ovarian drilling is followed, at least temporarily, by a high rate of spontaneous ovulation and conception, and that subsequent medical ovulation induction becomes easier. An analysis of 35 studies claims that 82% of women ovulated after LOD and 63% conceived spontaneously or after ovarian stimulation after LOD[30].

The Cochrane collaboration published a meta-analysis of six randomized high-quality trials of 15 available randomized trials in the literature[37]. There was no evidence of a difference in live births or ongoing pregnancies between LOD and gonadotropins. Multiple pregnancy rates were lower with ovarian drilling than with gonadotropins (1% vs. 16%, odds ratio (OR) 0.13, 95% confidence interval (CI) 0.03, 0.59). There was no evidence of a difference in miscarriage rates between the two groups (OR 0.81, 95% CI 0.36, 1.86).

Laparoscopic treatment of intra-abdominal adhesions

Intra-abdominal adhesions have been traditionally considered a cause of bowel obstruction, abdominal pain, pelvic pain and infertility. The etiological role of intra-abdominal adhesions in these circumstances, however, is not well documented. Of note, adhesions are usually not described as an etiological factor for pelvic pain in men. This might be related to a gender difference in pain perception or the possibility that adhesions *per se* do not cause pain. In addition, the efficacy, complication rates and recurrence rates of removing intra-abdominal adhesions are not well documented.

Endometriosis and intra-abdominal adhesions are the most common laparoscopic findings in patients with pelvic pain. Immunohistological studies have also shown evidence of nerve fibers in adhesions that had been removed from patients with and without pelvic pain. The cause of adhesion formation is unclear, but surgical procedures, local infections and genetic susceptibility have been suggested as being involved[38,39].

Numerous surgical techniques of adhesion removal have been described with markedly varying results. Authors have described outcomes of surgical adhesiolysis ranging from no pain relief to pain relief in 90% of patients. However, randomized trials to date have shown that adhesiolysis is ineffective in improving the outcome of the treatment of pelvic pain, possibly because of adhesion reformation[40].

Laparoscopic myomectomy

Uterine leiomyomas are associated with menorrhagia, dysmenorrhea and pelvic pressure. The role of uterine myomas as etiological factors of infertility is controversial. Specifically, the efficacy of surgical removal of myomas is debatable. Thus, the indication to remove myomas in infertility patients without clinical symptoms must be evaluated carefully.

There are many ways for myomas to impair fertility, including distortion of the uterine cavity, obstruction of the tubal ostia and alterations in the endometrium affecting embryo implantation and growth. However, because the incidence of uterine leiomyomas increases with age, fertility declines with age and many women with fibroids conceive spontaneously, it is difficult to assess the direct impact of leiomyomas on fertility. The American Society for Reproductive Medicine recommends myomectomy only after a complete evaluation of other potential factors for infertility[41].

Leiomyomas may be removed by hysteroscopy, laparotomy and laparoscopy. Laparoscopic myomectomy has been established as an appropriate alternative to abdominal myomectomy, hysterectomy and uterine artery embolization. Given an adequate level of specialization, laparoscopic myomectomy is superior to laparotomy for myoma removal. Results from randomized trials and clinical series demonstrated that laparoscopic myomectomy provides the advantages of shorter hospitalization, faster recovery, fewer adhesions and less blood loss than abdominal myomectomy when performed by skilled surgeons. Improvements in surgical instruments and techniques allows for safe intra-abdominal morcellation of the myoma and multilayer myometrial repair[42].

Removal of submucous and intramural myomas seems to be an effective method to achieve high pregnancy rates in infertility patients. A review of 23 studies on leiomyomas and reproduction reported an overall conception rate of 57% after myomectomy among prospective studies[43]. Among women with otherwise unexplained infertility, the conception rate was 61% after myomectomy. Studies cite uterine rupture rates after laparoscopic myomectomy of between 1 and 3%[44]. Recommendations for the duration of the time period to the next pregnancy vary between 3 and 12 months. There are no data establishing a recommendable interval between myoma removal and next pregnancy. In extrapolating from data about repeat cesarean sections, however, one can assume that a latency period of less than 18 months may increase the risk of uterine rupture[45].

The rate of cesarean section is significantly increased in women after myomectomy and is in the range of 70–80%[46].

Randomized trials support the use of absorbable adhesion barriers to reduce adhesions, but there is no apparent benefit of presurgical use of GnRH agonists[42].

In women with submucous myomas and infertility, hysteroscopic resection is the method of choice. Hysteroscopic myoma removal is safe and has acceptable rates of subsequent pregnancies. Vercellini *et al.* reported a series of 108 infertility patients[47]. The 3-year cumulative probability of conception was 49% in women with pedunculated lesions, 36% in those with sessile lesions and 33% in those with intramural lesions. In another series of women treated with hysteroscopic myoma removal, Fernandez *et al.* found that the procedure was most effective in terms of pregnancy rates when the removed myoma was the exclusive cause of infertility (pregnancy rate of 41.6%), and when the lesion was ≥ 50 mm in size (pregnancy rate of 57.1%)[48].

Assessment of Fallopian tube patency

The assessment of Fallopian tubes is crucial in the management of infertility, as approximately 30% of infertile patients are affected by tubal problems. If the diagnosis of Fallopian tube obstruction is missed the couple might be undergoing completely inefficient treatments. This creates frustration and results in wastage of resources. If the diagnosis of bilateral Fallopian tube obstruction is established the decision has to be taken whether a surgical procedure is indicated and, if it is, what the chances of success for this procedure are. These decisions should be left to specialists who have long-standing experience in this type of operation and who would counsel the patient, taking into consideration all relevant prognostic factors such as:

- Type of obstruction (distal or proximal)

- Cause of obstruction (iatrogenic due to sterilization procedure or endogenous due to infection)

- History of the patient, age of the patient and results of the patient's partner (if the partner has severely impaired semen quality, an operation is not indicated, as assisted reproductive technology (ART) is needed primarily).

For assessment of Fallopian tube patency several methods are available:

- Laparoscopy

- Hysterosalpingography (HSG)

- Hysterosalpingocontrast sonography (HyCoSy)

Laparoscopy

Laparoscopy can still be seen as the gold standard for assessment of tubal patency. In addition to evaluation of the tube, this method allows complete assessment of the pelvic structures. Visualization of the pelvic cavity is necessary to exclude or verify adnexal adhesions, endometriosis and other conditions that could interfere with ovum retrieval or negatively affect the outcome of treatment. Laparoscopy should be performed only if necessary interventions can be performed at the same time, e.g. adhesiolysis, salpingotomy, ovarian cystectomy or cauterization, or vaporization of endometriotic implants. This requires careful planning of experienced personnel and of equipment. It is a condition *sine qua non* that a surgeon performing laparoscopy should be able – at any time – to switch to open surgery (laparotomy) if required. This has to be considered when counseling the patient.

For assessment of tubal patency laparoscopy is performed under general anesthesia. Transcervical injection of methylene blue dye is performed and flow of the solution through the Fallopian tubes into the pelvic cavity is monitored (Figure 3.15). In this way a tubal obstruction can clearly be identified and the exact localization of the obstruction can be documented. If a distal obstruction is identified the decision must be taken as to whether a salpingostomy should be performed. If wide parts of the tube are destroyed due to chronic infection and adhesions/scars, etc. can be seen, a surgical reconstruction of 'normal anatomy' does not usually make sense as the indication is for IVF/ICSI.

In some cases the flow of methylene blue is very slow or heavy pressure must be exerted in order to pass the tubes. This can be interpreted as an impairment of tubal patency due to intratubal adhesions, scar tissue or other pathologies and – again – a surgical reconstruction is not indicated but the indication is for ART.

Hysterosalpingography

HSG is still the most widely used test of tubal patency. The advantage of HSG is that it allows simultaneous assessment of tubal patency and the uterine cavity. In comparative studies a good correlation between hystero-scopic findings and HSG results has been shown. HSG can detect fibroids, polyps and synechiae at a reasonable sensitivity and specificity. However,

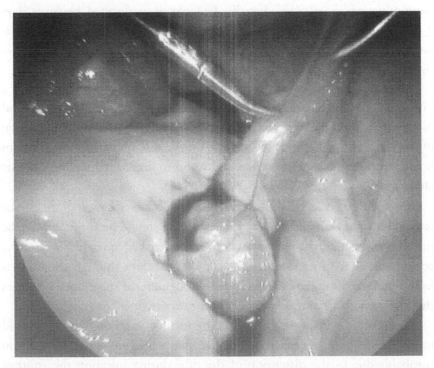

Figure 3.15   (See also Color Plate 4) Laparoscopic assessment of tubal patency: extrusion of the methylene blue solution through the distal end of the right tube is clearly visible

intrauterine synechiae and adhesions are not necessarily detected. The sensitivity and specificity for diagnosing tubal obstruction has been reported to be 65% and 83%, respectively.

The disadvantages of this method include a weakness in detecting peri-tubal adhesions, the necessity to use X-ray technique and the fact that in contrast to laparoscopy or HyCoSy (see below) it is a static procedure. Furthermore, many women find this procedure uncomfortable. HSG leads to unpleasant sensations especially in cases with tubal obstruction. Therefore, prostaglandin inhibitors could be administered 1–2 hours prior to the procedure.

Hysterosalpingocontrast sonography

Whereas in the past HSG was the standard first-line procedure for assessment of tubal patency, nowadays HyCoSy is increasingly being used. Tubal patency is assessed by transcervical injection of a water-soluble contrast medium while performing transvaginal ultrasound examination.

The contrast medium used for this investigation is a galactose solution containing micro-particles. Usually HyCoSy is performed between days 8–13 of the menstrual cycle, as during this time cervical catherization is facilitated due to the physiological opening of the cervix. Prior to the investigation a bacterial vaginal infection should be excluded.

At the beginning of the investigation the vagina is disinfected and a HyCoSy catheter (charière 5) is introduced into the uterine cavity and blocked thereafter. Most investigators start the investigation on visualization of the longitudinal view of the uterus. A small amount of contrast medium is injected to visualize the uterine cavity and to detect/exclude intrauterine abnormalities (Figure 3.16).

Once the uterine cavity has been studied, a transverse view of the uterus is achieved. The transverse layer of investigation should be at the level of the tubes to ensure that the media flow can be detected adequately. Some of the contrast medium is injected and the flow of medium through the tubes is followed. If the flow can be determined throughout the tubes until it reaches the free pelvic cavity, tubal patency can be expected.

Potential side-effects of the procedure include vasovagal reactions, mild to moderate pain, especially in those patients with tubal obstruction (probably due to the distension of the tube during injection the contrast medium) and in some cases nausea.

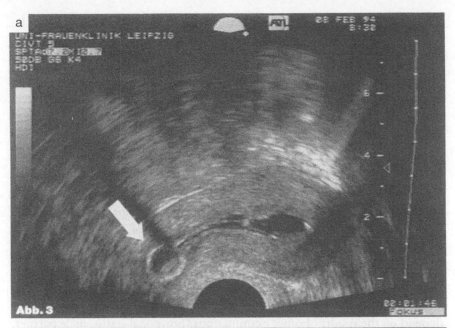

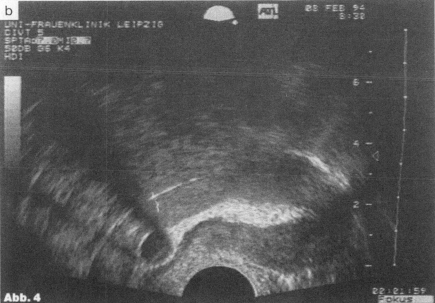

Figure 3.16 Longitudinal view of the uterus after insertion of the catheter (a). The correct localization of the balloon is confirmed (arrow). Afterwards a small amount of contrast medium is injected and the uterine cavity is assessed (b)

As for all other methods false-positive and -negative results have to be expected under certain conditions. In general, studies conducted to date have suggested that the sensitivity and specificity of HyCoSy is at least as good as for HSG. Therefore, taking into consideration that HSG X-ray technique has to be used and, furthermore, that HyCoSy is comparatively easier to perform, most units currently prefer HyCoSy as the first-line diagnostic procedure (Figure 3.17).

To increase the sensitivity/specificity further some groups applied Doppler ultrasound in conjunction with HyCoSy. It could be demonstrated that Doppler ultrasound optimizes visualization of the distal tubal portion and overall the concordance between HyCoSy and laparoscopy could be improved. However, at the same time routine use of Doppler ultrasound with HyCoSy certainly increases the complexity and the resources needed for this intervention, and therefore Doppler ultrasound is not routinely performed with HyCoSy.

If tubal patency can clearly be demonstrated, further treatment options depend on the results of other examinations (hormonal status, male partner, etc.). If results of the HyCoSy procedure cannot be interpreted properly or if there are remaining doubts on the integrity of pelvic structures,

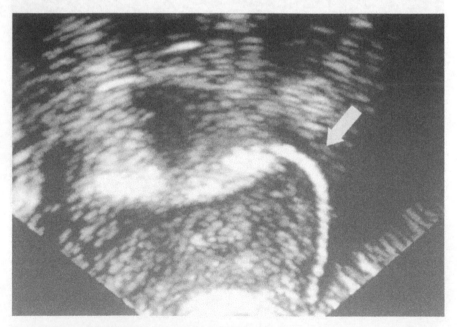

Figure 3.17 Assessment of tubal patency by hysterosalpingocontrast sonography. Constant flow of the contrast medium through the left tube

Table 3.5 Advantages and disadvantages of methods used for assessment of tubal patency

	Advantages	Disadvantages
Laparoscopy	Direct visualization of pelvic organs and the pelvic cavity; optimal assessment of tubo-ovarian contact; possibility to perform interventions	More invasive procedure due to general anesthesia and the surgical approach; requires more infrastructure and more resources; cost-intensive compared with the other procedures
HSG	Can be performed as an outpatient procedure; at the same time assessment of Fallopian tubes and uterine cavity	Patient is exposed to X-rays; risk of reaction to the contrast medium; no assessment of pelvic structures
HyCoSy	'Real-time' assessment of uterine cavity and tubal patency; can be performed as an outpatient procedure; anesthesia not necessary; relatively cheap	Distal portion of the tubes sometimes difficult to assess; galactosemia is a contraindication for the procedure

laparoscopy has to be performed to establish the diagnosis. The advantages and disadvantages of methods used for assessment of tubal patency are shown in Table 3.5.

REFERENCES

1. Bergmann MM, Jacobs EJ, Hoffmann K, Boeing H. Agreement of self-reported medical history: comparison of an in-person interview with a self-administered questionnaire. Eur J Epidemiol 2004; 19: 411–16
2. World Health Organization. Laboratory Manual for the Examination of Human Semen and Sperm–cervical Mucus Interaction, 4th edn. New York: Cambridge University Press, 1999
3. Menkveld R, Kruger TF. Advantages of strict (Tygerberg) criteria for evaluation of sperm morphology. Int J Androl 1995; 18 (Suppl 2): 36–42
4. Bals-Pratsch M, Knuth UA, Honigl W, et al. Pulsatile GnRH-therapy in oligozoospermic men does not improve seminal parameters despite decreased FSH levels. Clin Endocrinol 1989; 30: 549–60
5. Liu PY, Handelsman DJ. The present and future state of hormonal treatment for male infertility. Hum Reprod Update 2003; 9: 9–23

6. Glezermann M, Huleihel M, Lunenfeld E, et al. Efficacy of kallikrein in the treatment of oligozoospermia and asthenozoospermia: a double-blind trial. Fertil Steril 1993; 60: 1052–6

7. Keck C, Behre HM, Jockenhovel F, Nieschlag E. Ineffectiveness of kallikrein in treatment of idiopathic male infertility: a double-blind, randomized, placebo-controlled trial. Hum Reprod 1994; 9: 325–9

8. Pasquali R, Pelusi C, Genghini S, et al. Obesity and reproductive disorders in women. Hum Reprod Update 2003; 9: 359–72

9. Institute of Medicine, National Academy of Sciences. Nutrition during pregnancy. Washington, DC: National Academy Press, 1990

10. Torstveit MK, Sundgot-Borgen J. Participation in leanness sports but not training volume is associated with menstrual dysfunction: a national survey of 1276 elite athletes and controls. Br J Sports Med 2005; 39: 141–7

11. Crosignani PG, Colombo M, Vegetti W, et al. Overweight and obese anovulatory patients with polycystic ovaries: parallel improvements in anthropometric indices, ovarian physiology and fertility rate induced by diet. Hum Reprod 2003; 18: 1928–32

12. Hoeger KM, Kochman L, Wixom N, et al. A randomized, 48-week, placebo-controlled trial of intensive lifestyle modification and/or metformin therapy in overweight women with polycystic ovary syndrome: a pilot study. Fertil Steril 2004; 82: 421–9

13. Uchida S, Noda E, Kakazu Y, et al. Allopregnanolone enhancement of GABAergic transmission in rat medial preoptic area neurons. Am J Physiol Endocrinol Metab 2002; 283: E1257–65

14. Lang Dunlop A, Schultz R, Frank E. Interpretation of the BBT chart: using the 'Gap' technique compared to the Coverline technique. Contraception 2005; 71: 188–92

15. Baumann JE. Basal body temperature: unreliable method of ovulation detection. Fertil Steril 1981; 36: 729–33

16. Guermandi E, Vegetti W, Bianchi MM, et al. Reliability of ovulation tests in infertile women. Obstet Gynecol 2001; 97: 92–6

17. Lolarga E. A second look at natural family planning. Initiatives Popul 1983; 7: 2–12

18. Knochenhauer ES, Key TJ, Kashar-Miller M, et al. Prevalence of the polycystic ovary syndrome in unselected black and white women of the southeastern United States: a prospective study. J Clin Endocrinol Metab 1998; 83: 3078–82

19. Reindollar RH, Novak M, Tho SP, McDonough PG. Adult-onset amenorrhea: a study of 262 patients. Am J Obstet Gynecol 1986; 155: 531–43

20. Revised 2003 consensus on diagnostic criteria and long-term health risks related to polycystic ovary syndrome (PCOS). Hum Reprod 2004; 19: 41–7

21. Vermeulen A, Verdonck L, Kaufman JM. A critical evaluation of simple methods for the estimation of free testosterone in serum. J Clin Endocrinol Metab 1999; 84: 3666–72

22. Schiettecatte J, Van Opdenbosch A, Anckaert E, et al. Immunoprecipitation for rapid detection of macroprolactin in the form of prolactin–immunoglobulin complexes. Clin Chem 2005; 51: 1746–8

23. Fahie-Wilson MN, Ahlquist JA. Hyperprolactinaemia due to macroprolactins: some progress but still a problem. Clin Endocrinol 2003; 58: 683–5

24. Speroff L, Fritz MA, Amenorrhea. In Speroff L, Fritz MA, eds. Clinical Gynecologic Endocrinology and Infertility. Philadelphia: Lippincott Williams & Wilkins, 2005: 401

25. Freundl G, Tigges J. Gynäkologische Endokrinologie für die Praxis. Jena: Gustav Fischer Verlag, 1995

26. Rossmanith WG. Störungen des Prolaktinhaushalts. In Leidenberger F, Strowitzki T, Ortmann O, eds. Klinische Endokrinologie für Frauenärzte. Heidelberg: Springer Medizin Verlag, 2005: 301
27. Bakalov VK, Anasti JN, Calis KA, et al. Autoimmune oophoritis as a mechanism of follicular dysfunction in women with 46,XX spontaneous premature ovarian failure. Fertil Steril 2005; 84: 958–65
28. Lucisano A, Morandotti G, Marana R, et al. Chlamydial genital infections and laparoscopic findings in infertile women. Eur J Epidemiol 1992; 8: 645–9
29. Erel CT, Senturk LM. Is laparoscopy necessary before assisted reproductive technology? Curr Opin Obstet Gynecol 2005; 17: 243–8
30. Farquhar CM. The role of ovarian surgery in polycystic ovary syndrome. Best Pract Res Clin Obstet Gynaecol 2004; 18: 789–802
31. Donesky BW, Adashi EY. Surgical ovulation induction: the role of ovarian diathermy in polycystic ovary syndrome. Baillières Clin Endocrinol Metab 1996; 10: 293–309
32. Tasaka K, Sakata M, Kurachi H, et al. Electrocautery in polycystic ovary syndrome. Horm Res 1990; 33 (Suppl 2): 40–2
33. Liguori G, Tolino A, Moccia G, et al. Laparoscopic ovarian treatment in infertile patients with polycystic ovarian syndrome (PCOS): endocrine changes and clinical outcome. Gynecol Endocrinol 1996; 10: 257–64
34. Gjonnaess H. Late endocrine effects of ovarian electrocautery in women with polycystic ovary syndrome. Fertil Steril 1998; 69: 697–701
35. Farquhar CM. An economic evaluation of laparoscopic ovarian diathermy versus gonadotrophin therapy for women with clomiphene citrate-resistant polycystic ovarian syndrome. Curr Opin Obstet Gynecol 2005; 17: 347–53
36. Pirwany I, Tulandi T. Laparoscopic treatment of polycystic ovaries: is it time to relinquish the procedure? Fertil Steril 2003; 80: 241–51
37. Farquhar C, Lilford RJ, Marjoribanks J, Vandekerckhove P. Laparoscopic 'drilling' by diathermy or laser for ovulation induction in anovulatory polycystic ovary syndrome. Cochrane Database Syst Rev 2005; (3): CD001122
38. Wieser F, Tempfer C, Schneeberger C, et al. Interleukin-1 receptor antagonist polymorphism in women with peritoneal adhesions. Br J Obstet Gynaecol 2002; 109: 1298–300
39. Roberts LM, Sanfilippo JS, Raab S. Effects of laparoscopic lavage on adhesion formation and peritoneum in an animal model of pelvic inflammatory disease. J Am Assoc Gynecol Laparosc 2002; 9: 503–7
40. Hammoud A, Gago LA, Diamond MP. Adhesions in patients with chronic pelvic pain: a role for adhesiolysis? Fertil Steril 2004; 82: 1483–91
41. American Society for Reproductive Medicine Practice Committee. Myomas and reproductive function. American Society for Reproductive Medicine Practice Committee Report, November, 2001
42. Hurst BS, Matthews ML, Marshburn PB. Laparoscopic myomectomy for symptomatic uterine myomas. Fertil Steril 2005; 83: 1–23
43. Vercellini O, De Giorgi G, Aimi S, et al. Abdominal myomectomy for infertility: a comprehensive review. Hum Reprod 1998; 13: 873–9
44. Dubuisson JB, Fauconnier A, Deffarges JV, et al. Pregnancy outcome and deliveries following laparoscopic myomectomy. Hum Reprod 2000; 15: 869–73
45. Shipp TD, Zelop CM, Repke JT, et al. Interdelivery interval and risk of symptomatic uterine rupture. Obstet Gynecol 2001; 97: 175–7
46. Seracchioli R, Rossi S, Govoni F, et al. Fertility and obstetric outcome after laparoscopic myomectomy of large myomata: a randomized comparison with abdominal myomectomy. Hum Reprod 2000; 15: 2663–8

47. Vercellini P, Zaina B, Yaylayan L, et al. Hysteroscopic myomectomy: long-term effects on menstrual pattern and fertility. Obstet Gynecol 1999; 94: 341–7

48. Fernandez H, Sefrioui O, Virelizier C, et al. Hysteroscopic resection of submucosal myomas in patients with infertility. Hum Reprod 2001; 16: 1489–92

4

Pathology
4.1 Ovarian insufficiency

OVARIAN INSUFFICIENCY: WHO GROUPS I–IV

All women who enter menopause experience amenorrhea unless they receive hormone replacement therapy (HRT). In premenopausal women, amenorrhea unrelated to pregnancy, lactation, or drug interventions such as continuous progestogens or gonadotropin releasing hormone (GnRH) analogs, is a pathological phenomenon with implications for fertility, psychological health and bone stability. Amenorrhea may be the manifesting feature of a wide array of anatomic and endocrine abnormalities. Amenorrhea can occur as primary amenorrhea, i.e. with no history of menstruation, or as secondary amenorrhea, i.e. with a history of menstruation. The four most common causes of primary amenorrhea are:

• Ovarian failure (48.5%)

• Congenital absence of the uterus and vagina (16.2%)

• GnRH deficiency (8.3%)

• Constitutional delay of puberty (6.0%)[1]

In order to classify the various causes of secondary anovulation, the World Health Organization (WHO) has established a widely used classification. This classification comprises different subgroups of ovarian insufficiency and is considered by many experts to be a useful tool in clinical practice to establish the cause of secondary amenorrhea. Numerous scientific reports and treatment algorithms use this scheme and it is therefore advisable for physicians who are involved in the care of infertility patients to be familiar with the WHO classification.

Ovarian insufficiency: WHO group I – hypothalamic–pituitary failure

Anovulation and amenorrhea due to WHO group I ovarian insufficiency is caused by low concentrations of gonadotropins, i.e. follicle stimulating hormone (FSH), luteinizing hormone (LH), or both. This gonadotropin deficiency results in a lack of follicle development and follicular estrogen production. The term hypogonadotropic hypogonadism refers to the low levels of both pituitary gonadotropins and ovarian steroids.

There are many conditions resulting in reduced secretion of LH and FSH in the pituitary. Most commonly, marked weight loss secondary to starvation, a rigorous diet, or specific disorders such as anorexia nervosa can cause WHO group I ovarian insufficiency. The mechanistic link between weight loss and pituitary function is unclear. It has been proposed that the adipocyte-derived hormone leptin may be involved. Studies in animals and humans have demonstrated that low concentrations of leptin are fully or partly responsible for starvation-induced changes in neuroendocrine axes, including low reproductive, thyroid and insulin-like growth factor (IGF) hormones. In addition, exercise-induced hypothalamic amenorrhea and anorexia nervosa are also associated with low concentrations of leptin and a similar spectrum of neuroendocrine abnormalities[2].

As mentioned above, another reason for reduced pituitary gonadotropin secretion is physical stress. Sustained exercise programs such as those followed by professional athletes may result in anovulation and amenorrhea due to WHO group I ovarian insufficiency. Again, the biochemical link between physical stress and pituitary function is unknown, but low concentrations of leptin may be involved. In concordance with that hypothesis, leptin administration for the relative leptin deficiency in women with exercise-induced WHO group I ovarian insufficiency has been shown to restore ovulation, improve reproductive, thyroid and growth hormone axes and markers of bone formation[3]. These data suggest that leptin, a peripheral signal reflecting the adequacy of energy stores, is required for normal reproductive and neuroendocrine functions.

Isolated ('idiopathic') hypogonadotropic hypogonadism (IHH) is characterized by complete or partial failure of pubertal development due to impaired secretion of LH and FSH. A rare hereditary syndrome characterized by anosmia in combination with IHH and WHO group I ovarian failure is Kallmann's syndrome. Kallmann's syndrome has a molecular basis, as it may be caused by mutations of the X-chromosomal

KAL1 (encoding anosmin) or the fibroblast growth factor receptor 1 genes (FGFR1), both leading to agenesis of olfactory and GnRH-secreting neurons[4].

Iatrogenic damage to the pituitary gland may also result in local functional deficiencies and WHO group I ovarian insufficiency. This situation may occur after hypophysectomy or irradiation treatment for pituitary tumors. Another rare cause of pituitary damage and loss of function is severe postpartum hemorrhage. This condition is called Sheehan's syndrome. Clinically significant Sheehan's syndrome, however, is an uncommon consequence of obstetric hemorrhage in today's environment. In a study of 109 women with a history of obstetric hemorrhage, 14 complained of symptoms suggesting Sheehan's syndrome, e.g. menstrual dysfunction, lactation difficulty, cold intolerance, fatigue, axillary and pubic hair loss, and secondary infertility. None of these women, however, had abnormal levels of IGF-I, thyroxine (T4), prolactin (PRL), or early morning cortisol[5].

Ovarian insufficiency: WHO group II – hypothalamic–pituitary dysfunction

This group comprises by far the largest group of women affected by oligo- or anovulation. WHO group II ovarian insufficiency is characterized by normal concentrations of FSH and estradiol. Women falling into this group have an intact hypothalamus and pituitary, the pituitary–gonadal axis is functional, and ovarian steroids are produced. It is hypothesized that the synchronization of the various elements involved in the co-ordination of ovulation is deficient. For example, pathological timing of the pulsatile secretion of LH and FSH, androgen excess, or elevated concentrations of insulin are believed to cause a disruption of the pituitary–gonadal axis.

Around two-thirds of women with WHO group II ovarian insufficiency will be diagnosed with polycystic ovary syndrome (PCOS). This disorder is characterized by a combination of (1) oligo- or anovulation; (2) clinical and/or biochemical hyperandrogenism; and (3) ultrasonographic evidence of polycystic ovaries. Following a European Society for Human Reproduction (ESHRE) consensus definition, at least two of these three criteria must be present to establish a diagnosis of PCOS[6]. It is of note, that polycystic ovaries need not be present to make a diagnosis of PCOS and, conversely, their presence alone does not establish the diagnosis.

The definition of the above-mentioned diagnostic criteria is as follows:

- *Oligo-ovulation, anovulation*: oligo-ovulation is defined as ovulation frequency between 35 and 180 days or fewer than nine menses per year; anovulation is defined as no ovulation for at least 6 months

- *Hyperandrogenism*: clinical signs are hirsutism, acne, alopecia, virilization; biochemical signs are elevated serum concentrations of testosterone, androstenedione and/or the free testosterone index

- *Polycystic ovaries*: ultrasonographic evidence of at least 12 follicles with a diameter of < 10 mm

The etiology of PCOS is only partly understood. Many features of this syndrome are secondary to hyperandrogenemia, but a single cause of PCOS has not been identified. Because women with PCOS appear to have an increased LH pulse frequency, it has been speculated that the pulse frequency of GnRH is accelerated in the syndrome. It is not clear whether this accelerated pulse frequency is due to an intrinsic abnormality in the GnRH pulse generator or whether it is caused by the relatively low levels of progesterone resulting from infrequent ovulatory events. Since progestins slow the GnRH pulse generator down, low circulating progestin levels in women with PCOS may lead to an acceleration in the pulsatility of GnRH, increased levels of LH and overproduction of ovarian androgen.

Another characteristic feature of PCOS, although not included in the diagnostic algorithms, is peripheral insulin resistance. Women with PCOS have a greater frequency and higher degree of both hyperinsulinemia and insulin resistance than weight-matched controls. Of note, insulin resistance is, in principle, independent of obesity. Both lean and obese women with PCOS have evidence of decreased insulin sensitivity; however, insulin resistance is most marked where there is an interaction between obesity and the syndrome.

PCOS is associated with an approximately 35% decrease in insulin action, independent of the effect of obesity, which produces a close to 50% decrease in insulin action[7]. Insulin resistance has been increasingly recognized as an important feature of PCOS, being present in 50–70% of cases[8]. Insulin plays both direct and indirect roles in the pathogenesis of hyperandrogenemia in PCOS. Insulin acts synergistically with LH to enhance the androgen production of theca cells. Insulin also inhibits hepatic synthesis of sex hormone-binding globulin, the key circulating protein that binds to testosterone, and thus increases the proportion of testosterone that circulates in the unbound, biologically available, or free, state.

The relationship between hyperinsulinemia and PCOS has gained a great deal of attention in recent years, because a series of insulin-sensitizing agents have been shown to have therapeutic value in women with PCOS, among them metformin, troglitazone, rosiglitazone, pioglitazone and D-chiro-inositol. In a Cochrane review of 13 randomized controlled trials, metformin has been shown to be more effective than placebo, achieving ovulation in 76% and 46% of women when used with or without clomiphene, respectively[9]. Based on these data, metformin is now established as one option for first-line therapy in women with PCOS.

There is controversy over whether or not every woman with PCOS should be screened for glucose intolerance. The efficacy of insulin-sensitizing agents is independent of the presence of a pathological oral glucose intolerance test. Thus, this test should not be used for triaging women with PCOS in terms of treatment with metformin[3]. This recommendation is based on the observation that the clinical response to insulin-sensitizing agents is not related to the magnitude of insulin resistance. Also, insulin resistance is virtually universal and maximal once the body mass index (BMI) (defined as the weight in kilograms divided by the square of the height in meters) exceeds 30. Thus, there appears to be little value gained by formal measurement of insulin sensitivity in obese patients. Finally, it is important to note that readily available methods to quantify insulin resistance may be misleading, since they have been shown to lack precision when compared with the gold-standard method for quantifying whole-body insulin resistance, i.e. the hyperinsulinemic–euglycemic clamp.

On the other hand, screening may be useful to identify women with previously unknown diabetes and those at an elevated risk of developing type 2 diabetes in later life to enable them to have access to adequate prevention strategies. Screening is supported by evidence that the combined prevalence of impaired glucose tolerance and type 2 diabetes approaches 45% by the fourth decade, that both impaired glucose tolerance and type 2 diabetes are associated with significant morbidity, and that there is a substantial rate of conversion from impaired glucose tolerance to diabetes in the absence of intervention among women with PCOS. The American Diabetes Association recognizes PCOS as a risk factor that justifies screening for type 2 diabetes[10]. In our institution, we screen all women with PCOS using an oral glucose tolerance test. Aside from scientific interest, we believe that a pathological oral glucose tolerance test increases the patient's compliance with treatment recommendations, especially weight reduction. This claim, however, has not been validated in a properly designed study.

Several conditions have to be acknowledged when considering the differential diagnosis of PCOS in women with WHO group II ovarian insufficiency:

• Androgen-producing ovarian tumor

• 21-hydroxylase deficiency

• Cushing's syndrome

High serum concentrations of testosterone and a rapid onset of symptoms are indicative of an androgen-producing ovarian tumor. High serum concentrations of 17-hydroxyprogesterone are found in late-onset adrenal hyperplasia. The most common form of this disorder is 21-hydroxylase deficiency. These diagnoses, however, are rare. In a series of 201 women with hirsutism, one case of Cushing's syndrome, one case of androgen-producing ovarian tumor and two cases of 21-hydroxylase deficiency were identified[11]. In adrenogenital syndrome, sequence analysis of the steroid 21-hydroxylase gene has become an important tool to confirm or exclude suspected late-onset forms of the disease, where hormone measurements are not informative. Other causes of late-onset adrenogenital syndrome such as 11β-hydroxylase deficiency are rare. Nevertheless, accurate diagnosis of these often mild types of hyperandrogenism is important, since simple cortisol treatment can improve the clinical condition considerably.

Ovarian insufficiency: WHO group III – ovarian failure

This group of women is characterized by amenorrhea and hypergonadotropic hypogonadism, i.e. low serum concentrations of estradiol and high serum concentrations of FSH. The ovaries do not respond to the gonadotropic stimulus, owing to the lack of an ovarian reserve. In women with WHO group III ovarian failure, only a few follicles and oocytes or no follicles at all are found in the ovary. Reasons for ovarian failure include:

• Natural menopause

• Premature ovarian failure (POF)

• Chromosomal anomalies

Natural menopause occurs at a median age of 52 years and is defined as the last menstrual period with no menstrual period in the following year. Natural menopause occurs when the follicle pool is depleted. The number of ovarian follicles, available for menstrual recruitment between menarche and menopause, is defined by the size of the primordial follicle pool. This pool is established during the fetal period with a peak of 6–7 million at 20 weeks' gestation and subsequently reduced by follicle atresia to approximately 1–2 million oocytes at birth and 300 000 at the time of puberty. The threshold number of follicles at the time of menopause is estimated to be around 1000[12].

The timing of menopause has a high degree of variability and a wide variety of factors are believed to influence the duration of the reproductive lifespan. Epidemiological studies found environmental, lifestyle and anthropometric factors to be associated with the number of lifetime menstrual cycles and the duration of the reproductive lifespan, among them smoking, nulliparity, oral contraceptive use, early surgical removal of one ovary, a history of depression, and irregularity and duration of menstrual bleeding[13].

Furthermore, a strong genetic contribution to the duration of the reproductive lifespan has been documented in twin studies and sib-pair analyses with heritability estimates of 0.71 and 0.87 for affected sisters and twins, respectively[14].

Generally, cessation of menses before the age of 40 is termed POF although some authors define POF as the cessation of menses even before the age of 35. POF has a strong genetic component and shows familial clustering. Mutations of several genes such as the FSH receptor gene or the galactose-1-phosphate uridyl transferase gene as well as autoimmune oophoritis have been cited as possible etiological factors in women with POF[15].

POF is not a definitive state, since approximately 5–10% of women with a diagnosis of POF may conceive spontaneously and unexpectedly after the diagnosis. This has to be kept in mind when discussing the diagnosis with affected women.

In a longitudinal monocenter study, 18 out of 30 000 patients were diagnosed as having primary amenorrhea. Six had primary amenorrhea due to chromosomal aberrations. The most common cause was Turner's syndrome seen in four out of six[16]. Other chromosomal anomalies may also occasionally be found, e.g. 45,X/46,XX mosaicism.

Ovarian insufficiency: WHO group IV – hyperprolactinemia

Hyperprolactinemia, defined as elevated PRL levels (> 20 µg/l) found on at least two occasions, is a common finding in clinical endocrinology. Hyperprolactinemia is the most common endocrine disorder of the hypothalamic–pituitary axis. Characteristic symptoms include amenorrhea or oligomenorrhea, galactorrhea and infertility. Patients may also present with osteopenia and cumulative effects of a pituitary tumor. The frequency of galactorrhea in women with hyperprolactinemia has been reported as ranging from 30 to 83%. There are several possible causes of hyperprolactinemia, among them autonomous production in the pituitary, medication that alters the inhibitory actions of dopamine and primary hypothyroidism.

Drugs associated with hyperprolactinemia are those that reduce central dopamine neurotransmission by blocking dopamine receptors (e.g. phenothiazines, butyrophenones, metoclopramide) or those depleting central catecholamine stores (e.g. reserpine). Other drugs that can result in hyperprolactinemia include tricyclic antidepressants, opiates, verapamil and large parenteral doses of cimetidine.

Hyperprolactinemia may also be caused by non-hypothalamic–pituitary disease. For example, 40% of patients with primary hypothyroidism have mild elevation of PRL levels that can be normalized by treatment of the underlying condition. Therefore, assessment of thyroid hormones, i.e. triiodothyronine (T3), T4 and thyroid stimulating hormone (TSH), should be included in the routine diagnostic work-up of a patient with hyperprolactinemia. About 30% of patients with chronic renal failure and up to 80% of patients on hemodialysis also have elevated PRL levels. This is probably secondary to decreased clearance and increased production of PRL as a result of disordered hypothalamic regulation of prolactin secretion. Correction of the renal failure by transplantation results in normoprolactinemia.

Since pituitary adenomas are a possible cause of hyperprolactinemia, one aim of the diagnostic algorithm is to rule out a PRL-producing pituitary adenoma which may or may not compress the pituitary stalk. Owing to the anatomic proximity of the sella turcica to the chiasma opticum, visual disturbance may occur as a clinical symptom of a prolactinoma.

Elevated serum concentrations of PRL are found during pregnancy and lactation. During normal pregnancy, the serum PRL level rises progressively to around 200–500 ng/ml (4000–10 000 mU/l), an increase thought to be due to rising estrogen concentrations. If pregnancy and lactation are ruled out, the likelihood of a prolactinoma is significantly increased with values > 50 µg/l and relatively certain with values between 200 µg/l and 500 µg/l[17]. On these occasions or if the patient complains about visual disturbances, a magnetic resonance imaging (MRI) scan of the sella region is recommended. Rarely, prolactin concentrations of > 1000 µg/l are found, which is indicative of an invasive prolactinoma.

In a series of 271 women with hyperprolactinemia, Berinder *et al.* found oligomenorrhea or amenorrhea in 87% of the women of reproductive age; 47% had galactorrhea. Microadenomas were found in 63%, macroadenomas in 8% and idiopathic hyperprolactinemia in 29%. Interestingly, they found no differences in PRL levels between patients with or without galactorrhea[18].

Some patients have an apparently high PRL level without any clinical features of hyperprolactinemia. This may be caused by 'big' prolactin or macroprolactin, representing dimers, trimers or polymers of prolactin, or prolactin–immunoglobulin immune complexes. Such forms are rarely physiologically active but may register in certain prolactin assays. Thus, differentiation between prolactin and 'big' prolactin variants has to be discussed with the laboratory at each individual institution.

A useful diagnostic algorithm facilitating a rapid diagnosis and treatment starts with:

(1) Prolactin – confirming/ruling out WHO group IV;

(2) Estradiol – confirming WHO group II, if normal;

(3) FSH – ruling out WHO group I, if low and confirming WHO group III, if high.

4.2 Hyperandrogenemia

Androgen excess in women can be derived from the ovary, the adrenal glands, or the peripheral conversion of androgen precursors. The most common cause of androgen excess is polycystic ovary syndrome (PCOS). PCOS has been discussed previously.

Less frequent causes of hyperandrogenism are 21-hydroxylase-deficient non-classical adrenal hyperplasia, the hyperandrogenic insulin-resistant acanthosis nigricans syndrome, androgen-secreting tumors and androgenic drug intake. Also, idiopathic hyperandrogenemia may occur, which is in most cases associated with obesity. The increased aromatase (CYP 19) activity and hyperinsulinemia observed in obese women are believed to play a major role in causing hyperandrogenemia, either by stimulating LH secretion or by direct stimulation of the ovary. In addition to ovarian hyperandrogenemia, hypothalamic–pituitary dysfunction has been observed in response to obesity. Inadequate central serotonin stimulation, excessive dopamine stimulation and insensitivity to endorphins may all be involved in pituitary–hypothalamic dysfunction[19].

Table 4.1 lists conditions other than PCOS, which may be considered in women with hyperandrogenemia.

A baseline testosterone level higher than 7 nmol/l makes functional hyperandrogenism highly unlikely and points towards tumorous hyperandrogenism. Testosterone levels below 4.5 nmol/l were not seen in ovarian tumors secreting androgens in a series of 38 hyperandrogenic women who failed to respond to an oral 2-mg 48-hour low-dose dexamethasone suppression test[21].

Among the less common causes of hyperandrogenism, ovarian and adrenal tumors are the most challenging in terms of establishing a diagnosis.

Table 4.1 Conditions associated with hyperandrogenemia

Condition	Hyperandrogenemia, hyperandrogenism or both	Oligomenorrhea or amenorrhea	Distinguishing features	
			Clinical	Hormonal or biochemical
Non-classic congenital adrenal hyperplasia due to deficiency of 21-hydroxylase	Yes	Not often	Family history of infertility, hirsutism or both; common in Ashkenasi Jews	Elevated (basal) level of 17-hydroxyprogesterone in the morning or on stimulation
Cushing's syndrome	Yes	Yes	Hypertension, striae, easy bruising	Elevated 24-hour urinary free cortisol level
Hyperprolactinemia or prolactinoma	None or mild	Yes	Galactorrhea	Elevated plasma prolactin level
Primary hypothyroidism	None or mild	May be present	Goiter may be present	Elevated plasma thyrotropin and subnormal plasma thyroxine level; prolactin level may also be increased
Acromegaly	None or mild	Often	Acral enlargement, coarse features, prognathism	Increased plasma insulin-like growth factor I
Premature ovarian failure	None	Yes	May be associated with other autoimmune endocrinopathies	Elevated plasma follicle stimulating hormone and normal or subnormal estradiol level
Simple obesity	Often	Not often	Diagnosed by exclusion	None
Virilizing adrenal or ovarian neoplasm	Yes	Yes	Clitoromegaly, extreme hirsutism, or male-pattern alopecia	Extremely elevated plasma androgen level
Drug-related condition*	Often	Variably	Evidence provided by history	None

*A drug-related condition is a condition due to the use of androgens, valproic acid, cyclosporine or other drugs

Although rare exceptions do exist, suppression of the elevated androgen levels following the administration of dexamethasone excludes the presence of an autonomous functioning adrenal tumor[22]. Furthermore, the ovarian contribution to androgen secretion in women with hyperandrogenism is affected by the administration of dexamethasone, suggesting that dexamethasone responsiveness can be used to exclude autonomous androgen secretion. The ovarian component to the hyperandrogenism can also be assessed by evaluating the degree of androgen suppression to estrogen or GnRH-analog administration; however, several gonadotropin-dependent ovarian steroid-secreting tumors have been described. Although imaging techniques, particularly ultrasonography and computed tomography (CT), have been extensively used to demonstrate adrenal or ovarian pathology in hyperandrogenic women, they may fail to localize ovarian tumors which are small and embedded within the ovary. MRI is an alternative imaging technique, and has been found to be useful in this context[23]. Invasive techniques have also been used to identify the presence of ovarian androgen-producing tumors by biochemical analysis of blood obtained from the adrenal and ovarian veins during venous catheterization[24].

Of patients with androgen excess, 70–80% demonstrate hirsutism[25]. Conversely, not all hirsute patients have evidence of detectable androgen excess, as 5–15% of these women have 'idiopathic hirsutism', with normal ovulatory function and androgen levels.

4.3 Endometriosis

INTRODUCTION

Endometriosis is a common estrogen-dependent benign disease. It is characterized by the presence of uterine endometrial tissue outside the normal location – mainly on the pelvic peritoneum, but also on the ovaries and other pelvic organs. In rare cases endometrial tissue can also be found in extrapelvic locations such as the pericardium, the pleura and even in the brain. Data on the incidence of endometriosis are sometimes conflicting as they vary with different definitions and different methods for detection of endometriosis: in some papers the incidence of endometriosis is calculated on the basis of 'typical clinical symptoms' whereas others classify the disease on the basis of laparoscopic findings.

In the general population the prevalence of pelvic endometriosis is reported to be 6–10%, whereas in populations with pain, infertility or both, the frequency is 35–50%.

Theories of pathogenesis

Over the years different theories have been developed to explain the pathogenesis of endometriosis (Table 4.2).

Independent of what theory is applied, there seem to be mechanisms that are crucial for the disease to be established:

- Attachment of endometrial tissue to the peritoneum

- Invasion of the endothelium and establishment of blood supply

Table 4.2 Different theories on the pathogenesis of endometriosis
Retrograde menstruation
Metaplasia of peritoneal cells
Alteration of local immunological environment
Genetic origin
Environmental factors
Multifactorial: interaction between specific genes and environmental factors

• Establishment of a specific local environment to prevent 'clearance' of the dystopic endometrial tissue from the peritoneum

The most widely accepted theory is that the disorder originates from retrograde menstruation. This theory is supported by the finding that women suffering from endometriosis reveal higher volumes of menstrual blood reflux. Furthermore, these women show a different pattern of myometrial contractility: subendometrial myometrial contractile waves are more frequent compared with healthy controls. The risk for development of endometriosis is higher for women with primary amenorrhea due to cervical obstruction and in animal models it has been shown that endometriosis can be induced in baboons by ligation of the cervix. One factor, which challenges the retrograde menstruation theory, is that most women have some degree of retrograde menstruation but only 6–10% have endometriosis.

The metaplasia theory claims that endometriosis is induced by metaplasia of the celomic epithelium under the influence of environmental factors and on the basis of a specific genetic profile of the affected patients.

Genetic factors

Most of the theories mentioned above claim that patients with endometriosis need to have a specific genetic background. The concept of endometriosis as an inheritable disease is supported by the fact that the risk of developing the disease for first-degree relatives of women with severe endometriosis is six-fold higher than in the normal population. Furthermore, familial aggregation has been confirmed in large population-based studies and twin-studies. Currently, linkage studies are being performed applying a genome-wide search for polymorphisms to identify candidate genes for endometriosis. Findings reported so far indicate that mutations and polymorphisms in detoxification enzymes might be a common finding in endometriosis patients, which could lead to an increased susceptibility to environmental toxins. Furthermore, it has been shown that polymorphisms in tumor suppressor genes are more frequent in women with endometriosis compared with normal controls. This finding would support the metaplasia theory. A genetic database for the epidemiology of endometriosis has been established and can be screened for further information (http://www.well.ox.ac.uk/krinaz/genepi_endo.htm).

Immunological factors

Besides genetic factors, immunological factors seem to be involved in the pathogenesis of endometriosis. In particular, mechanisms involved in the local immune response seem to be different in women suffering from endometriosis compared with controls. Thus, it has been shown that peritoneal macrophages of women with endometriosis secrete more cytokines as well as a different pattern of cytokines compared with macrophages from unaffected controls. Furthermore, macrophages from endometriosis patients show a decreased phagocytic activity, which explains why the peritoneal cavity is not 'cleared' of dystopic endometrial tissue. Cells isolated from endometriotic lesions as well as peritoneal cells of endometriosis patients secrete factors that interact with the local cytokine metabolism. Thereby, the secretion of interleukins, growth factors and angiogenic factors is significantly increased and elevated concentrations of these factors can be found in peritoneal fluid. It has been postulated that the elevated concentrations of these factors in peritoneal fluid are not only a result of endometriotic lesions but can actively promote growth and activity of dystopic endometrial cells. These findings are the basis of therapeutic concepts, which try to block the cytokine cascades and thereby try to interrupt the vicious circle between endometriotic lesions–cytokine secretion–growth and activity of dystopic endometrium.

Some authors claim that endometriosis is an autoimmune disease. This hypothesis is based on increased polyclonal B cell activity, abnormalities in function of B and T cells, familial inheritance, high B cell and T cell counts and reduced natural killer cell activity. Furthermore, high serum concentrations of IgG, IgA and IgM autoantibodies as well as antiendometrium antibodies have been reported for endometriosis patients. Women with endometriosis reveal a significantly increased risk for autoimmune and endocrine disorders such as fibromyalgia, chronic fatigue syndrome, systemic lupus erythematosus, etc. This should be considered for the diagnostic work-up of endometriosis patients.

Environmental factors

As mentioned above some theories on the pathogenesis of endometriosis claim that environmental factors play a key role. In animal models it has been shown that exposure to whole-body proton irradiation increases the risk for endometriosis. Furthermore, chronic exposure to dioxin in rhesus monkeys resulted in a dose-dependent increase of endometriosis. This fits with the epidemiological finding that Belgium, with the highest dioxin pollution in the world, has the highest incidence of endometriosis as well as the highest prevalence of severe endometriosis.

As endometriosis is an estrogen-dependent disease, environmental factors associated with estrogenic effects have been extensively studied. However, to date there has been no epidemiological study definitely linking one class of chemicals to the risk of endometriosis. This lack of a definitive link is not surprising, because people are exposed to a multiplicity of chemicals with mechanisms of action that might vary with dose, timing of exposure, route of exposure and synergy with other chemicals. In summary, to date environmental factors cannot be ruled out as contributing to the development of endometriosis. However, a clear link between individual factors or individual classes of factors and the development of endometriosis has not yet been established.

ENDOMETRIOSIS AND INFERTILITY

Studies in animal models as well as in patients claim that endometriosis as such has a negative impact on fertility. This seems to be true for the situation of spontaneous conception as well as for assisted conception. Results for assisted reproductive technology (ART) registers reveal that pregnancy rates (PR) in patients with endometriosis are significantly lower compared with those of patients with tubal disease. In properly controlled studies the association between endometriosis and the following parameters has been established:

- Poor ovarian reserve

- Low oocyte and embryo quality

- Poor implantation rate

It seems obvious that adhesions and other anatomical abnormalities, which might be induced by endometriosis, impair the fertility potential of women affected by endometriosis. However, results of recent research indicated that peritoneal fluid from women with endometriosis with high concentrations of cytokines, growth factors and activated macrophages exerts toxic effects on sperm function and embryo survival. In different animal models it has been shown that this peritoneal fluid also impairs implantation rates in rabbits, mice and hamsters. It has clearly been shown that women with severe endometriosis reveal different gene expression as well as differences in eutopic and dystopic endometrium.

Women with endometriosis – once achieving a pregnancy – reveal a much higher incidence of the following complications during pregnancy:

- Pregnancy loss

- Preterm delivery

- Intrauterine growth restriction

- Pre-eclampsia

It is speculative whether these adverse outcomes are the results of a suboptimal implantation process or of immune dysfunction in women with endometriosis. However, awareness of potential complications is needed in women with known endometriosis once a pregnancy is achieved.

From what has been said so far it is evident that the association between endometriosis and infertility cannot be established on the basis of a single pathogenetic factor; it is rather a complex interaction of pathogenetic variables and an individual disposition for development of the disease.

ENDOMETRIOSIS AND LOCAL ESTROGEN METABOLISM

As endometriosis is an estrogen-dependent disease, much attention has been paid to the local regulation of estrogen metabolism. It has been shown that endometriotic lesions show higher estradiol biosynthesis and lower estradiol inactivation compared with endometrium from unaffected women. Therefore, many treatment strategies for endometriosis are based on a reduction of endogenous estradiol production.

Aromatase

Although the ovary and the adrenal gland are the main sources of endogenous estrogens, several human tissues and organs are capable of estrogen production, provided they express aromatase. Aromatase is the key enzyme for endogenous estrogen production as it catalyzes the conversion of androstenedione and testosterone derived from ovarian and adrenal sources to estrone and estradiol, respectively. In premenopausal women, ovarian granulosa cells represent the primary site of aromatase expression. Therefore, ovarian secretion accounts for the largest portion of estradiol production in women in the reproductive age group. Aromatase expression in the ovary is mainly regulated by FSH, which activates a signaling pathway involving cyclic adenosine monophosphate (cAMP) steroidogenic factor-1 (SF-1) and cAMP response element binding protein (CREB). Binding of the two latter factors to the promoter of the CYP 19 (aromatase P450) gene gives rise to the events leading to the production of aromatase protein.

In postmenopausal women – after cessation of ovarian function – extraovarian tissues become the major source of estrogen production. Aromatase activity is especially high in adipose tissue.

Physiologically, uterine tissues do not produce estrogens. However, it has been shown that CYP 19 gene expression and aromatase activity can be found in uterine leiomyomas, endometrial cancer and endometriosis. It is intriguing that these are all estrogen-dependent conditions. Therefore, it can be concluded that aromatase activity is absent in disease-free uterine tissue, whereas aromatase expression is inappropriately activated in estrogen-dependent disorders of the uterus such as endometriosis.

Several groups have shown that aromatase expression is much higher in endometriotic tissue compared with adipose tissue and that endometriotic stromal cells are the primary source of aromatase. Furthermore, it has been demonstrated that aromatase expression can be regulated locally by various factors among which prostaglandins play a major role. In particular, PGE_2 significantly induced aromatase expression. From this mechanism the vicious circle becomes obvious: endometriotic lesions produce significant amounts of prostaglandins and thereby augment endogenous estrogen production, which in turn stimulates activity of the endometriotic lesion.

The pathophysiological mechanisms outlined above provide the basis for treatment of endometriosis with aromatase inhibitors, which will be discussed below.

DIAGNOSIS AND TREATMENT OF ENDOMETRIOSIS

To establish the diagnosis of endometriosis, ultrasound examinations or laparoscopy might be applied. The diagnostic value of different methods is shown in Table 4.3.

In many cases patients report the typical ('classical') symptoms of endometriosis:

• Pelvic pain

• Dysmenorrhea

• Dyspareunia

Therefore, if patients report one or more of these symptoms, the diagnosis 'endometriosis' is likely. However, in some cases, even if none of these symptoms is reported, extensive endometriotic plaques can be detected at laparoscopy and vice versa. Even if all these symptoms are reported, laparoscopy does not necessarily reveal findings that correlate with severe endometriosis.

If endometriosis affects the ovary and leads to the typical chocolate cyst this can easily be detected on ultrasound, owing to the typical structure of these cysts. However, in cases without cysts but massive adhesions/plaques elsewhere in the pelvis, ultrasound fails to confirm the diagnosis, therefore the diagnostic value is limited.

Serum markers such as CA125 or PP14 are positively correlated with endometriosis. However, they are very unspecific and therefore their diagnostic value is very low.

Table 4.3 Diagnostic value of different methods/measurements

Method/marker	Diagnostic value
History	+
Gynecological examination	+/−
Ultrasound examination	+/−
Serum CA125 / PP 14	−
Laparoscopy	+++

−, low; +++, very high

Laparoscopy is currently seen as the gold standard for diagnosis of endometriosis, for several reasons:

(1) Only by laparoscopy can a complete evaluation of the pelvic and abdominal cavity be achieved;

(2) Plaques and adhesions which are not detectable on ultrasound can easily be detected and classified by laparoscopy;

(3) The extent of endometriosis (number of lesions, diameter of lesions, etc.) can be evaluated only by laparoscopy;

(4) To establish the diagnosis firmly, histology of the lesions should be examined. This can easily be done by laparoscopy;

(5) During laparoscopy tubal patency can be tested and thereby important information can be gained;

(6) If endometriosis is diagnosed, surgical treatment of the lesions can be performed at the same time.

Of course, the same aspects as mentioned above for laparoscopy can be achieved by conventional laparotomy. However, today laparoscopy is seen as first-line surgical treatment of endometriosis and only in rare cases is open laparotomy necessary.

Figures 4.1–4.5 show 'classical examples' of laparoscopic findings in patients with endometriosis.

CLASSIFICATION OF ENDOMETRIOSIS

Different scoring systems have been developed to classify and stage endometriosis. The most widely used classification is that proposed by the American Fertility Society (ASRM classification; www.asrm.org/literature/classifications/classification.html). Another classification which is predominantly used in Europe is the Endoscopic Endometriosis Classification (EEC) (Figure 4.6).

The systems mentioned above are morphology based and classify endometriosis on the basis of the number, localization and diameter of lesions. The ASRM system, in particular, is limited in that it is designed to predict only the likelihood of future fertility. There is no correlation between the stage of disease and the degree of pain or the prognosis with treatment.

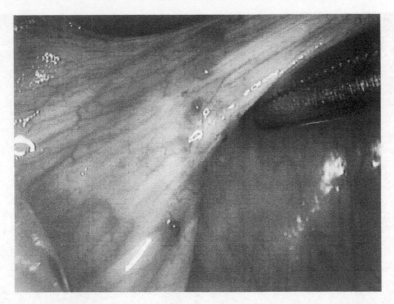

Figure 4.1 (See also Color Plate 5) Minimal endometriosis at the uterine ligaments in a 23-year-old patient without clinical symptoms

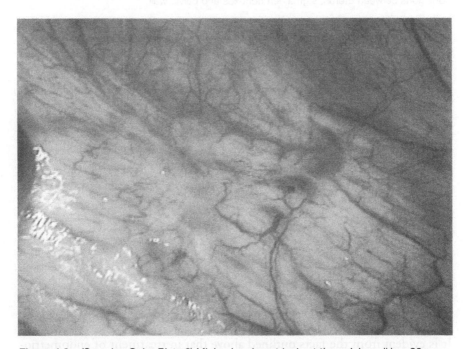

Figure 4.2 (See also Color Plate 6) Minimal endometriosis at the pelvic wall in a 30-year-old patient without symptoms

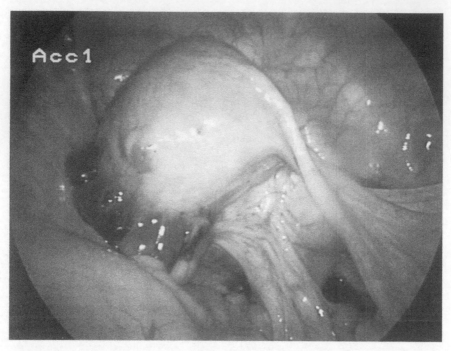

Figure 4.3 (See also Color Plate 7) Massive endometriosis in a 24-year-old patient with adhesions between uterus, sigma, left adnexes and pelvic wall

As pain is one of the most dominant symptoms of clinically relevant endometriosis, the disease can – besides the ASRM and EEC classification – be graded according to the American Fertility Society by the respective level of pain caused by the lesions:

- A: mild

- B: discomforting

- C: distressing

- D: horrible

- E: excruciating

TREATMENT PRINCIPLES OF ENDOMETRIOSIS

It is evident from the facts outlined above that in treatment of endometriosis we deal with different entities. Surgical treatment of endometriosis is still

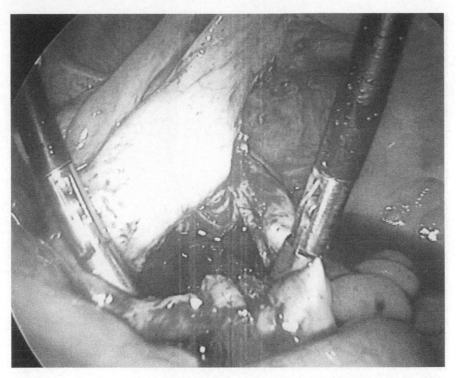

Figure 4.4 (See also Color Plate 8) Chocolate cyst of the left ovary. Surgical removal of the cyst

the gold standard. However, the question of whether primary surgery or primary medical treatment should be performed cannot be answered in a general way and for all scenarios.

- If endometriosis is diagnosed 'by chance' during a routine laparoscopy and the patient does not have any symptoms, surgery should be rather restrictive and would – besides other factors – depend on the specific experience of the surgeon.

- If the patient were undergoing the surgical procedure due to severe typical symptoms of endometriosis, the aim of the intervention would usually be to remove all endometriotic lesions that are visible – if this is possible from a surgical standpoint. This kind of procedure should be performed only in specialized centers where different disciplines with extensive experience in this kind of treatment are available.

- It is well known that endometriotic ovarian cysts (chocolate cysts) usually do not shrink adequately on medical treatment. Therefore, if a persistent

93

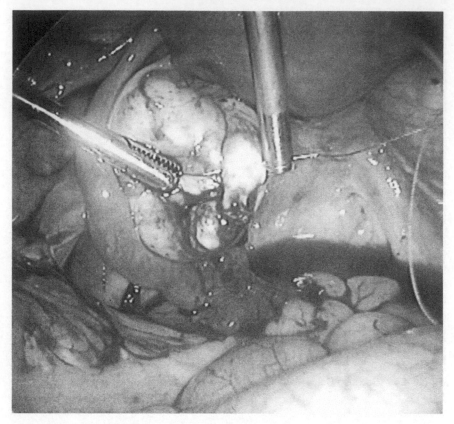

Figure 4.5 (See also Color Plate 9) Reconfiguration of the ovary after removal of the cyst

chocolate cyst is found with a diameter that causes a risk for the patient (torsion of the ovary) laparoscopic extirpation of the cyst is needed. There is no uniform recommendation on the threshold for the diameter of cysts that need intervention. However, most experts would anticipate a risk if the cyst persistently reveals a diameter of more than 10 cm whereas for cysts with a diameter of less than 4–5 cm usually an expectant approach is justified.

Besides the fundamental questions of surgical versus medical treatment, the treatment strategy also clearly depends on the major aim of treatment. One has to differentiate whether the treatment is directed at the endometriosis itself and its respective lesions, or if the treatment is directed at the symptoms caused by endometriosis: pain (dysmenorrheal, chronic pelvic pain, dyspareunia, pain at defecation, etc.) or infertility.

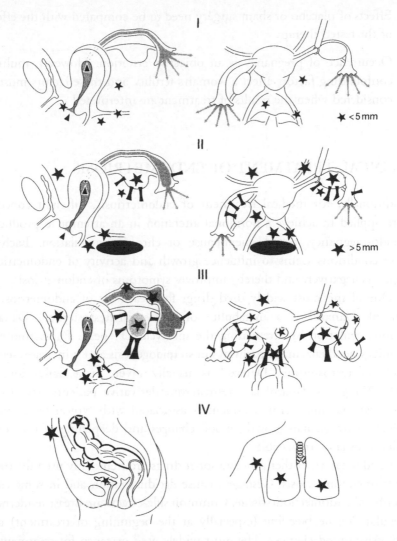

I

II

III

IV

★ <5 mm

★ >5 mm

Figure 4.6 Endometriosis classification according to the Endoscopic Endometriosis Classification

If efficacy of treatment is measured by assessing its effects on pain and infertility at the first moment, this seems to be easy. However, several factors have to be taken into consideration:

• A validated pain scale is needed

• A time-dependent evaluation is mandatory, as pain as well as infertility might vary depending on the observation period

- Effects of placebo or sham surgery need to be compared with the effects of the tested therapy

- Occurrence of pregnancy is an objective criterion. However, multiple confounding factors affect a woman's fertility and these factors must be considered when the results of treatment are interpreted

MEDICAL TREATMENT OF ENDOMETRIOSIS

Traditionally, for medical treatment of endometriosis, different concepts were applied to achieve a hormonal alteration in an attempt to produce a pseudo-pregnancy, pseudo-menopause or chronic anovulation. Each of these conditions seems to influence growth and activity of endometriotic implants negatively and thereby improves symptoms of endometriosis.

One of the most widely used drugs for treatment of endometriosis is danazol. Danazol is a metabolite of 17α-ethinyltestosterone. Danazol inhibits ovulation by attenuating the midcycle LH peak. Furthermore, it inhibits several enzymatic pathways in steroidogenesis and it increases serum levels of testosterone. Danazol is usually given at a daily dose of 600–800 mg. As danazol is a testosterone derivative patients have to be informed that long-term treatment is associated with typical testosterone effects: increased hair growth, mood changes and deepening of the voice, which is usually irreversible.

Besides danazol other progestational drugs are frequently used for treatment of endometriosis. Gestagens cause decidualization and in some cases atrophy of endometriotic tissue. Common side-effects are breast tenderness, irregular uterine bleeding (especially at the beginning of treatment) and depressive mood changes. The most widely used gestagen for treatment of endometriosis is medroxyprogesterone acetate (MPA), which is usually given at a dose of 20–30 mg/day. Some authors recommend doses up to 100 mg. Whereas MPA has to be administered daily, other gestagens such as gestrinone can be applied 2–3 times per week. Gestrinone has mild to moderate androgenic and antiestrogenic side-effects. As already mentioned for danazol, the patients have to be informed that some of these changes (deepening of the voice, clitoris hypertrophy) – although rare – might be irreversible.

A very common treatment (especially first-line treatment) of endometriosis is the use of a combination therapy with estrogens + progestins in the form of a contraceptive pill. The oral contraceptives (OCs) can be given cyclically or continuously. There is no proof that one or the other schedule has an advantage with respect to its effects on endometriotic lesions. However, especially women with severe dysmenorrhea seem to benefit from continuous treatment. Side-effects of OCs include weight gain, irregular bleeding (in the beginning) and, in rare cases, hypertension.

Whereas OCs, gestagens and danazol are usually applied as first-line therapy, GnRH agonists (GnRH-a) are seen as second-line treatment. GnRH-a decrease endogenous LH and FSH secretions and thereby induce a hypogonadotropic state. They can be applied intramuscularly, subcutaneously or intranasally and, depending on the GnRH-a used, application intervals range from daily to several months (usually 3 months for depot preparations). GnRH-a can induce the full picture of hypoestrogenism: hot flashes, vaginal dryness, decreased libido, depressive mood, fatigue, etc. Patients usually do not perceive these symptoms at the beginning of treatment but usually after treatment for 3 or more months.

To compensate for these side-effects, recently the so-called 'add-back' regimen was introduced. At the same time that GnRH-a are given, estrogens and progestogens are substituted at doses that are usually applied in HRT for postmenopausal symptoms. Thus, treatment efficacy of GnRH-a remains constant but most of the symptoms of hypoestrogenism can be eliminated.

If, due to treatment of endometriotic lesions, the endometriosis-related symptoms disappear, alternative/additional treatment options need not be sought. However, even if in most cases successful treatment of endometriotic lesions automatically leads to pain relief or to restoration of fertility, in other patients this is not the case so that treatment strategies have to be revised. GnRH-a as well as danazol have been shown successfully to relieve pain in endometriosis patients. Both drugs appear to be equally effective in this respect. If this treatment is not sufficient for pain relief, non-steroidal anti-inflammatory drugs (NSAIDs) have successfully been applied. NSAIDs significantly decrease production of prostaglandins in endometriotic lesions and thereby decrease pain.

The above-mentioned treatment concepts reveal some striking disadvantages. Even if successful inhibition of the pituitary–ovarian axis is achieved, a 100% response rate can never be expected. This is most probably due to the presence of estradiol production from the adipose tissue, skin and endometriotic lesions, which cannot be blocked by GnRH-a. All concepts introduced above are associated with 'iatrogenic infertility' as pregnancy does not occur in the hypoestrogenic state induced by either of the treatments.

These aspects provide the rationale to look for alternative approaches and try to develop medical treatments of endometriosis, which are not associated with the drawbacks mentioned.

Treatment of endometriosis by aromatase inhibitors

It has to be pointed out that currently aromatase inhibitors (AIs) are not registered for treatment of endometriosis. Therefore, the results referred to below derive from experimental studies performed under adequately controlled conditions. However, they cannot be transferred to the human situation directly.

The rationale for treatment of endometriosis with AIs is that blockade of aromatase activities in extraovarian sites might keep a larger proportion of patients in remission for a longer time. Furthermore, the application of AIs does not interfere with the physiological feedback mechanisms and therefore in principle under AI treatment pregnancies can occur. One of the first cases successfully treated with AIs was reported by Takayama et al.[26] in a 57-year-old postmenopausal patient with aggressive endometriosis which, even after hysterectomy and bilateral salpingo-oophorectomy, showed recurrence of the disease with severe pelvic pain and bilateral urethral obstruction leading to left kidney atrophy and right hydronephrosis. Treatment with gestagens was ineffective. After 1 month of treatment with anastrozole, significant pain relief and a regression of vaginal endometriotic lesions was observed. At the same time a reduction of serum estrogen levels could be detected as well as a decrease of aromatase expression in endometriotic lesions of this patient. Treatment with AIs might negatively affect bone density of the patients, therefore it might have to be combined with osteoprotective substances.

The above-mentioned case report was challenged, and a recent study by Ailawadi et al.[27] showed that premenopausal women who were resistant to other types of surgical or medical endometriosis therapy could successfully be treated by a combination of AIs and norethindrone acetate. The majority of patients had significant pain relief and endometriotic lesions clearly decreased in size and activity after a 6-month treatment.

In conclusion, although currently still experimental, aromatase inhibitors may represent a new generation of medications for the treatment of endometriosis as either first- or second-line treatment.

Treatment of endometriosis with tumor necrosis factor-α binding protein

Another experimental treatment for endometriosis, which might in the future become available, is treatment with tumor necrosis factor-α binding protein (TBP-1). It has been shown that tumor necrosis factor (TNF)α modulates cytokines and chemokines, which are associated with the inflammatory response of endometriosis. In animal models[28,29] it has been shown that treatment with the TNFα binding protein could significantly reduce endometriotic lesions and, furthermore, in baboons, it could prevent the occurrence of endometriotic implants and endometriosis-related adhesions. Treatment of endometriosis by TBP would in principle not interfere with the physiological feedback mechanisms and thereby proper control of endometriotic symptoms, so a pregnancy could be achieved.

It must be emphasized that the results referred to above are from animal studies and we must wait to see whether these results can be extended to the situation in the human.

Although this book mainly addresses conservative treatment, at least the basic principles of ART treatment for patients with endometriosis should be discussed, as this is a frequent disease and the practitioner will quite often be confronted with the questions of whether or not ART procedures should be applied primarily or secondarily.

Endometriosis and ovulation induction or intrauterine insemination

Ovulation induction in anovulatory patients as well as intrauterine insemination (IUI) in combination with mild ovarian stimulation (MOH) have been proved to be effective in certain groups of patients (see above). However, it is unclear whether patients with endometriosis benefit from these treatments.

Nuojua-Huttunen et al.[30] in a retrospective study compared success rates for IUI + MOH and showed that pregnancy rates were 6.5, 11.8 and 15.3% for patients with endometriosis, male factor infertility and unexplained infertility, respectively. These findings were confirmed in a prospective study by Omland et al.[31] showing 16.3 versus 33.6% pregnancy rates for patients with endometriosis and unexplained infertility, respectively, undergoing IUI with MOH. Hughes[32] showed that the diagnosis 'endometriosis' as such decreased per cycle conception rates in IUI + MOH protocols by half.

Endometriosis and ART

It has already been mentioned that there is no uniform therapeutic approach for endometriosis patients. This also applies to the application of ART for patients with endometriosis. In a young patient with mild endometriosis ART would probably be postponed until conservative treatment and IUI + MOH had been tried without achieving a pregnancy. In a woman of advanced reproductive age, ART techniques might be warranted more expeditiously, as with increasing age chances for conception drop significantly.

From the pathophysiology of endometriosis it can be concluded that the disease exerts negative effects on several crucial steps in the conception process: it has been demonstrated that endometriosis as such impairs implantation and early embryo development. Therefore, it can be speculated that the use of *in vitro* fertilization (IVF)/intracytoplasmic sperm injection (ICSI) procedures removes some of the critical steps such as fertilization and early embryo development from the *in vivo* situation to the 'safer' *in vitro* situation. However, it has been shown that endometriosis patients reveal significantly lower pregnancy rates in ART compared with other patient groups. Barnhart *et al.*[33] published a meta-analysis including 22 original articles on the outcome of ART in endometriosis patients and showed that patients with severe endometriosis had lower pregnancy rates, decreased fertilization and implantation rates and a decreased number of oocytes retrieved.

There is a difference between earlier studies and contemporary studies looking at the oocyte yield for patients with different grades of endometriosis. Whereas some older studies reported a lower number of oocytes retrieved in endometriosis patients[34,35], in modern treatment protocols using the transvaginal retrieval method and modern concepts of ovarian stimulation there does not seem to be a negative influence of endometriosis on the number of oocytes retrieved[36,37]. Furthermore, in a study by Olivennes *et al.*[38] it was confirmed that there was no correlation between the number of oocytes retrieved and the grade of the disease.

In modern ovarian stimulation protocols gonadotropins are usually combined with a GnRH-antagonist or GnRH-agonist (GnRH-a) for prevention of a premature LH surge. As GnRH-a are standard treatment for endometriosis it has been a matter of debate whether long- or short-term GnRH-a pretreatment should be used for ovarian stimulation of endometriosis patients. Nakamura *et al.*[39] compared GnRH-a suppression for 60 days with a shorter, midluteal down-regulation protocol and they reported 67 versus 27% pregnancy rates. This was confirmed by Marcus and Edwards[40], and Surrey et al.[41]. However, other authors could not confirm a difference between long and short GnRH-a pretreatments[42], therefore overall it appears that endometriosis patients behave similarly under ovarian stimulation compared with other patients. However, there is an overall tendency in the literature to show that longer GnRH-a protocols might provide an advantage.

Surgery and ART

Data concerning the benefit of surgery on the outcome of ART procedures are conflicting. There are few prospective randomized controlled trials available on this topic. Whereas Garcia-Velasco et al.[43] did not find any difference with or without surgery on IVF outcome in endometriosis patients, a recent Cochrane review[44] including two trials comparing the effectiveness of laparoscopic surgery versus other treatment modalities in endometriosis showed that laparoscopic surgery may improve the chance of pregnancy by an odds ratio of 1.6.

In summary, at the moment due to a lack of data no final conclusion can be drawn on whether surgery prior to ART significantly alters the results.

CONCLUSION

ART procedures in principle are no different for patients with or without endometriosis. However, in terms of ovarian stimulation there might be a difference for endometriosis patients. Whereas it has clearly been shown that GnRH-antagonists are as effective as agonists overall for ovarian stimulation, it seems as if endometriosis patients might gain a slight improvement from long-term agonist protocols. However, as for other questions, these need to be addressed by controlled prospective studies, which currently are not available.

The decision of conservative treatment versus ART for patients with endometriosis needs to be taken on an individual basis, as several patient-related factors have to be considered, among which patient age is one of the key factors. Whereas in young patients application of the available conservative treatment and IUI + MOH might be justified, for women of older reproductive age ART procedures should be offered earlier within the therapeutic cascade, as overall chances of conception significantly decrease with age.

4.4 Uterine fibroids

Uterine fibroids affect 20–50% of women of reproductive age, and the prevalence increases with age. Thus, uterine fibroids are the most common benign tumors in this population. Clearly, most cases of uterine fibroids have no clinical relevance, and the presence of uterine fibroids *per se* should not be an indication for medical or surgical intervention. It should be noted that the frequency of uterine fibroids is not increased in women with infertility: they are present in approximately 5–10% of women with infertility, and are the sole factor identified in 1–2.4% of these women[45]. Fibroids have been implicated in both recurrent pregnancy loss and infertility, but these associations are subject to debate. There is no consensus about the impact of uterine fibroids on fertility.

The rationale for an association between the presence of uterine fibroids and infertility comprises distortion of the uterine cavity, occlusion of the tubal ostia, altered uterine contractility, local inflammation and altered cytokine microenvironment[46]. Although these theories are plausible, there is no randomized clinical trial proving the efficacy of surgical removal of uterine fibroids with respect to infertility.

Several reviews summarized the evidence of retrospective and prospective, non-randomized trials in IVF couples and concluded that the presence of uterine fibroids negatively affects IVF outcome.

Pritts reviewed 11 IVF studies and noted that patients with submucosal fibroids and abnormal uterine cavities had significantly lower pregnancy rates (relative risk (RR) 0.32), implantation rates (RR 0.28) and delivery rates (RR 0.75) compared with infertile controls without fibroids[46]. It should be noted that infertile women with fibroids had significantly lower implantation rates than infertile controls, but only submucosal fibroids had a significant impact on pregnancy and delivery rates. These studies also demonstrated that pregnancy rates increased after myomectomy of submucosal fibroids. This meta-analysis therefore concluded that submucosal and intracavitary fibroids negatively affect reproductive outcomes and should therefore be removed, and that neither intramural nor subserosal fibroids adversely impact fertility.

Donnez and Jadoul summarized six studies looking at IVF outcomes in women with and without fibroids. They found a significant decrease in pregnancy rates when the uterine cavity was distorted compared with a non-distorted cavity and patients without fibroids (9% vs. 33.5% and 40%, respectively)[47]. The authors concluded that submucosal as well as intramural fibroids with a visible distortion of the uterine cavity based on ultrasound and/or hysteroscopy significantly impaired implantation and pregnancy rates in IVF patients.

In a third review of the literature, Surrey reviewed a number of studies to investigate the impact of intramural fibroids on IVF outcomes[48]. The author concluded that submucosal and intramural fibroids close to the endometrial cavity negatively impact IVF outcome and recommended surgical removal in these cases.

In a review of studies performed between 1990 and 2002, Benecke et al. investigated the impact of intramural leiomyomata on pregnancy outcome in assisted reproduction[49]. There was a significant negative impact on implantation rate in the intramural myomata groups versus the control groups (16.4 vs. 27.7%; odds ratio (OR) 0.62). The delivery rate per transfer cycle was also significantly lower (31.2 vs. 40.9%; OR 0.69). These data support the notion that patients with intramural fibroids have a lower implantation rate per cycle than patients without fibroids.

Whether or not myomas should be removed prophylactically, i.e. before a planned IVF, is controversial. Most authors, however, recommend surgical procedures only after one or more IVF failures. It is our practice, however, to decide this issue on an individual basis, especially if there is proven distortion of the uterine cavity.

Although several medical therapies may reduce fibroid volume or decrease menorrhagia, myomectomy remains the 'Gold Standard' treatment. It is important to note the high rates of recurrence after surgical removal of uterine fibroids. In a retrospective study of Japanese women, for example, transvaginal ultrasound examinations were performed in 135 women after abdominal myomectomy. The cumulative recurrence rates at 12 and 24 months were 12.4 and 46.0%, respectively[50]. Women with a history of

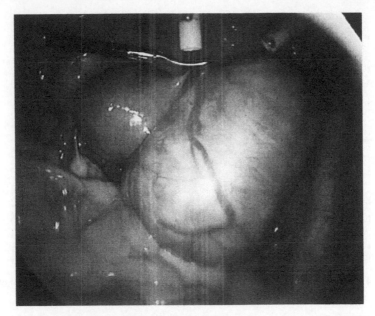

Figure 4.7 (See also Color Plate 10) Subserous fibroid in a 28-year-old woman with infertility for 3 years. Diameter of fibroid: 8 cm

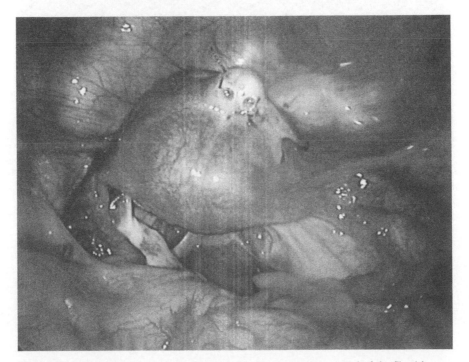

Figure 4.8 (See also Color Plate 11) Situs after laparoscopic removal of the fibroid

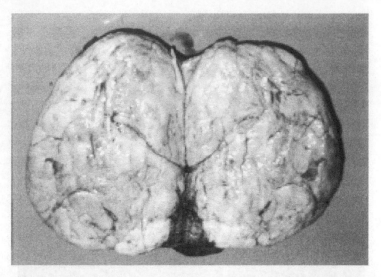

Figure 4.9   (See also Color Plate 12) Typical macroscopic aspect of fibroid morphology

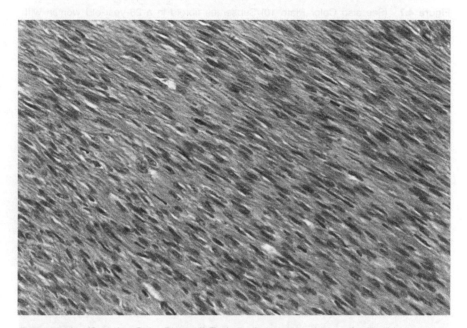

Figure 4.10   (See also Color Plate 13) Typical microscopic picture of a fibroid:
- Muscle fibers form vortex-like structures
- Ovoid or nearly rectangular nuclei
- Sometimes nuclei arranged in palisades
- Varying amount of collagen fibers

previous myomectomy and those with removal of four or more uterine fibroids had a significantly higher risk of recurrence.

Alternative methods of uterine fibroid removal in women with infertility include uterine artery embolization, uterine artery ligation, myolysis, laparoscopic coagulation and destruction of uterine fibroids.

Recent data identified an increased rate of pregnancy complications after uterine artery embolization compared with laparoscopic myomectomy. A new procedure, MRI-guided focused ultrasound ablation, shows promising results for the management of symptomatic fibroids, and possibly for the management of fibroids prior to pregnancy. For embolization and other alternative techniques, more data are needed to evaluate post-procedure fertility and pregnancy outcomes. In summary, these techniques are considered experimental and should not be offered to women with infertility outside clinical trials.

REFERENCES

1. Timmreck LS, Reindollar RH. Contemporary issues in primary amenorrhea. Obstet Gynecol Clin North Am 2003; 30: 287–302
2. Chan JL, Mantzoros CS. Role of leptin in energy-deprivation states: normal human physiology and clinical implications for hypothalamic amenorrhoea and anorexia nervosa. Lancet 2005; 366: 74–85
3. Welt CK, Chan JL, Bullen J, et al. Recombinant human leptin in women with hypothalamic amenorrhea. N Engl J Med 2004; 351: 987–97
4. Karges B, de Roux N. Molecular genetics of isolated hypogonadotropic hypogonadism and Kallmann syndrome. Endocr Dev 2005; 8: 67–80
5. Feinberg EC, Molitch ME, Endres LK, Peaceman AM. The incidence of Sheehan's syndrome after obstetric hemorrhage. Fertil Steril 2005; 84: 975–9
6. The Rotterdam ESHRE/ASRM-sponsored PCOS consensus workshop group. Revised 2003 consensus on diagnostic criteria and long-term health risks related to polycystic ovary syndrome (PCOS). Hum Reprod 2004; 19: 41–7
7. Dunaif A, Segal KR, Futterweit W, Dobrjansky A. Profound peripheral insulin resistance, independent of obesity, in polycystic ovary syndrome. Diabetes 1989; 38: 1165–74
8. Goodarzi MO, Korenman SG. The importance of insulin resistance in polycystic ovary syndrome. Fertil Steril 2003; 80: 255–8
9. Lord JM, Flight IH, Norman RJ. Insulin-sensitising drugs (metformin, troglitazone, rosiglitazone, pioglitazone, D-chiro-inositol) for polycystic ovary syndrome. Cochrane Database Syst Rev 2003; (3): CD003053
10. American Diabetes Association. Screening for type 2 diabetes. Diabetes Care 2004; 27 (Suppl 1): S11–S14
11. Glintborg D, Henriksen JE, Andersen M, et al. Prevalence of endocrine diseases and abnormal glucose tolerance tests in 340 Caucasian premenopausal women with hirsutism as the referral diagnosis. Fertil Steril 2004; 82: 1570–9

12. Gosden RG, Faddy MJ. Biological bases of premature ovarian failure. Reprod Fertil Dev 1998; 10: 73–8
13. Harlow BL, Signorello LB. Factors associated with early menopause. Maturitas 2000; 35: 3–9
14. de Bruin JP, Bovenhuis H, van Noord PAH, et al. The role of genetic factors in age at natural menopause. Hum Reprod 2001; 16: 2014–18
15. Nelson LM, Covington SN, Rebar RW. An update: spontaneous premature ovarian failure is not an early menopause. Fertil Steril 2005; 83: 1327–32
16. Jabbar S. Frequency of primary amenorrhea due to chromosomal aberration. J Coll Physicians Surg Pak 2004; 14: 329–32
17. Speroff L, Fritz MA. Amenorrhea. In Speroff L, Fritz MA, eds. Clinical Gynecologic Endocrinology and Infertility. Philadelphia: Lippincott Williams & Wilkins, 2005: 401
18. Berinder K, Stackenas I, Akre O, et al. Hyperprolactinaemia in 271 women: up to three decades of clinical follow-up. Clin Endocrinol (Oxf) 2005; 63: 450–5
19. Friedman CI, Kim MH. Obesity and its effect on reproductive function. Clin Obstet Gynecol 1985; 28: 645–63
20. Ehrmann DA. The polycystic ovary syndrome. N Engl J Med 2005; 352: 1223–36
21. Kaltsas GA, Mukherjee JJ, Kola B, et al. Is ovarian and adrenal venous catheterization and sampling helpful in the investigation of hyperandrogenic women? Clin Endocrinol (Oxf) 2003; 59: 34–43
22. Derksen J, Nagasser SK, Meinders AE, et al. Identification of virilizing adrenal tumours in hirsute women. N Engl J Med 1994: 331: 968–73
23. Outwater EK, Marchetto B, Wagner BJ. Virilizing tumors of the ovary: imaging features. Ultrasound Obstet Gynecol 2000; 15: 365–71
24. Loh KC, Lo JC, Zaloudek CJ, Fitzgerald PA. Occult virilizing ovarian tumors in post-menopausal women: problems in evaluation with reference to a case. Ann Acad Med Singapore 1988; 27: 712–16
25. Sanchez LA, Knochenhauer ES, Gatlin R, et al. Differential diagnosis of clinically evident hyperandrogenism: experience with over 1000 consecutive patients [Abstract]. Fertil Steril 2001; 76: S111
26. Takayama K, Zeitoun K, Gunby RT, et al. Treatment of severe postmenopausal endometriosis with an aromatase inhibitor. Fertil Steril 1998; 69: 709–13
27. Ailawadi RK, Jobanputra S, Kataria M, et al. Treatment of endometriosis and chronic pelvic pain with petrozole and norethindrone acetate: a pilot study. Fertil Steril 2004; 81: 290–6
28. Barrier BF. Efficacy of anti-tumor necrosis factor therapy in the treatment of spontaneous endometriosis in baboons. Fertil Steril 2004; 81 (Suppl 1): 775–9
29. D'Hooghe TM, Nugent NP, Cuneo S, et al. Recombinant human TNFRSF1A (r-hTBP1) inhibits the development of endometriosis in baboons: a prospective, randomized, placebo- and drug-controlled study. Biol Reprod 2006; 74: 131–6
30. Nuojua-Huttunen S, Tomas C, Bloigu R, et al. Intrauterine insemination treatment in subfertility: an analysis of factors affecting outcome. Hum Reprod 1999; 14: 698–703
31. Omland A, Tanbo T, Dale PO, Abyholm T. Artificial insemination by husband in unexplained infertility compared with infertility associated with peritoneal endometriosis. Hum Reprod 1998 13: 2602–5
32. Hughes EG. The effectiveness of ovulation induction and intrauterine insemination in the treatment of persistent infertility: a meta-analysis. Hum Reprod 1997; 12: 1865–72
33. Barnhart K, Dunsmoor-Su R, Coutifaris C. Effect of endometriosis on in vitro fertilization. Fertil Steril 2002; 77 1148–55

34. Chillik CF, Acosta AA, Garcia JE, et al. The role of in vitro fertilization in infertile patients with endometriosis. Fertil Steril 1985; 44: 56–61
35. Oehninger S. In vitro fertilization and embryo transfer (IVF/ET): an established and successful therapy for endometriosis. J In Vitro Fert Embryo Transf 1988; 5: 249–56
36. Dmowski WP, Rana N, Michalowska J, et al. The effect of endometriosis, its stage and activity and of autoantibodies on in vitro fertilization and embryo transfer success rates. Fertil Steril 1995; 63: 555–62
37. Bergendal A, Naffah S, Nagy C, et al. Outcome of IVF in patients with endometriosis in comparison with tubal-factor infertility. J Assist Reprod Genet 1998; 15: 530–4
38. Olivennes F, Feldber D, Liu HC, et al. Endometriosis: a stage by stage analysis – the role of in vitro fertilization. Fertil Steril 1995; 64: 392–8
39. Nakamura K, Oosawa M, Kondou I, et al. Metrodin stimulation after prolonged gonadotrophin releasing hormone agonist pretreatment for in vitro fertilization in patients with endometriosis. J Assist Reprod Genet 1992; 9: 113–17
40. Marcus SF, Edwards RG. High rates of pregnancy after long-term down-regulation of women with severe endometriosis. Am J Obstet Gynecol 1994; 171: 812–17
41. Surrey ES, Silverberg KM, Surrey MW, Schoolcraft WB. Effect of prolonged gonadotrophin-releasing hormone agonist therapy on the outcome of in vitro fertilization–embryo transfer in patients with endometriosis. Fertil Steril 2002; 78 699–704
42. Chedid S, Camus M, Smitz J, et al. Comparison among different ovarian stimulation regimens for assisted procreation procedures in patients with endometriosis. Hum Reprod 1995; 10: 2406–11
43. Garcia-Velasco JA, Mahutte NG, Corona J, et al. Should endometriomas be removed prior to IVF? Proceedings of the 58th Annual Meeting of the American Society of Reproductive Medicine, Seattle, WA, 2002
44. Jacobson T, Barlow D, Koninckx P, et al. Laparoscopic surgery for subfertility associated with endometriosis (Cochrane Review) In The Cochrane Library, Issue 1, 2004. Chichester, UK: John Wiley and Sons
45. Buttram VC, Reiter RC. Uterine leiomyomata: etiology, symptomatology, and management. Fertil Steril 1981; 36: 433–45
46. Pritts EA. Fibroids and infertility: a systematic review of the evidence. Obstet Gynecol Surv 2001; 56: 483–91
47. Donnez J, Jadoul P. What are the implications of myomas on fertility? A need for a debate? Hum Reprod 2002; 17: 1424–30
48. Surrey ES. Impact of intramural leiomyomata on in-vitro fertilization–embryo transfer cycle outcome. Curr Opin Obstet Gynecol 2003; 15: 239–42
49. Benecke C, Kruger TF, Siebert TI, et al. Effect of fibroids on fertility in patients undergoing assisted reproduction. A structured literature review. Gynecol Obstet Invest 2005; 59: 225–30
50. Nishiyama S, Saito M, Sato K, et al. High recurrence rate of uterine fibroids on transvaginal ultrasound after abdominal myomectomy in japanese women. Gynecol Obstet Invest 2006; 61: 155–9

5

Ovulation induction
5.1 Clomiphene citrate

INTRODUCTION

Clomiphene citrate (CC) has been used for induction of ovulation since 1961[1]. It was a breakthrough in the treatment of infertility associated with anovulation. After more than 40 years of clinical use, CC still appears to be quite useful, because it is orally administered and cheap compared with other drugs which are injected and more expensive. Furthermore, it is an effective medication. However, recent development of new oral medications such as aromatase inhibitors and insulin sensitizers has challenged the clinical use of CC in routine medical practice.

MECHANISMS OF ACTION

CC contains an unequal mixture of two isomers. Zyclomiphene is the most potent with a long half-life; however, it accounts for only 38% of the total drug content of each tablet.

As shown in Figure 5.1, CC has both estrogenic and antiestrogenic properties[2]. Acting as an antiestrogen, CC is thought to displace endogenous estrogen from hypothalamic estrogen receptor sites. Therefore, by blocking the negative feedback exerted by estrogen at the hypothalamic level, CC is able to restore pulsatile secretion of GnRH. Consequently, the subsequent increases in endogenous FSH and LH levels promote follicular growth and ovulation.

Furthermore, experimental data suggest that CC has an estrogenic, rather than an antiestrogenic, effect at the pituitary and ovarian levels which

111

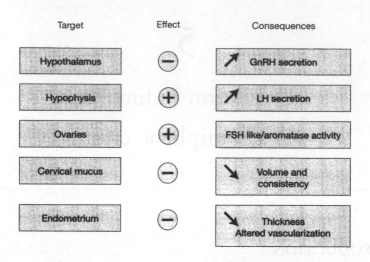

Target	Effect	Consequences

Figure 5.1 Antiestrogenic and estrogenic properties of clomiphene citrate with consequences on target tissues. GnRH, gonadotropin releasing hormone; LH, luteinizing hormone; FSH, follicle stimulating hormone

could amplify the action of this compound on the hypothalamic–hypophyseal–ovarian axis. Nevertheless, CC also acts as an antiestrogenic agent on cervical mucus and on the endometrium which may partly reduce the benefit of this preparation in terms of pregnancy rate. These data indicate the potential positive and negative effects of CC related to its estrogenic and antiestrogenic properties on different targets.

INDICATIONS

In accordance with its mechanism of action, any use of CC requires some degree of endogenous estrogen secretion and preserved ovarian function. Therefore, its main indication is ovulation induction for World Health Organization (WHO) group II anovulation, particularly when associated with polycystic ovary syndrome (PCOS). In this situation, CC is able to counteract the negative effect of estradiol which is presumably increased at the hypothalamic level.

The use of CC is also quite common for ovarian stimulation in unexplained infertility in order to boost ovulatory capacity in conjunction with intrauterine insemination (IUI).

PROTOCOLS

CC is administered orally, typically starting on day 2–5 after the onset of spontaneous or progestin-induced menses. The starting dose is usually a single tablet (50 mg) for 5 days with 50 mg increments in subsequent cycles until ovulation is induced. A meta-analysis of 13 studies[3] has recently reported that only 46% of the patients responded to 50 mg and that a larger dose of 100 and 150 mg was effective in 21% and 8% of patients, respectively. As doses in excess of 100 mg/day are not approved by the Food and Drug Administration (FDA), it has been suggested that a longer course (8 days) of CC treatment could be prescribed, but no benefit has been demonstrated so far.

MONITORING THE STIMULATION CYCLE

While CC has been prescribed without any monitoring for a long time, there is now compelling evidence that careful but not necessarily frequent monitoring of CC-treated cycles by ultrasound evaluation of follicular growth and endometrial thickness on day 12–14 of the cycle is justified, for several reasons:

- To identify patients who are not responding or have depressed endometrial thickness

- To detect those who over-respond and are exposed to the risk of multiple pregnancies

- To determine the timing of natural intercourse or IUI

Confirmation of ovulation is usually performed by basal body temperature chart or, more precisely, by measurement of serum progesterone levels in the assumed midluteal phase.

RESULTS AND OUTCOMES

A collection of published data has been recently presented[4]. Cumulative ovulation and pregnancy rates from 5268 patients showed an ovulation rate of 73% and pregnancy rate of 36% (Table 5.1)[5–11].These data are in accordance with those previously reported (ovulation rate of 60–85% and

	No. of patients	Ovulation	Pregnancy	Abortion	Live births
Table 5.1 Results of treatment with clomiphene citrate: a collection of published data. From reference 4					
McGregor et al. (1968)[5]	4098	2869	1393	279	1114
Garcia et al. (1977)[6]	159	130	64	16	48
Gysler et al. (1982)[7]	428	364	184	24	160
Hammond (1984)[8]	159	137	67	10	57
Kousta et al. (1997)[9]	128	113	55	13	42
Messinis et al. (1998)[10]	55	51	35	4	31
Imani et al. (2002)[11]	259	194	111	11	98
Total (% of patients)	5286 (100)	3858 (73)	1909 (36)	357 (7)	1550 (29)

pregnancy rate of 30–40%)[9,12]. Overall, the miscarriage rate is about 20% (between 13 and 25%). Multiple pregnancy rate is rarely addressed in published reports and estimates vary between 8 and 13%, the vast majority being twin pregnancies. There is no evidence that CC treatment increases the overall risk of birth defects.

PREDICTIVE FACTORS FOR A POSITIVE RESPONSE

Failure to ovulate (CC resistance)

Owing to the fact that 27% of patients remain anovulatory and about 64% of patients do not conceive following CC administration, the need to assess the predictive factors of CC response has recently been highlighted[13,14]. It has been shown that the probability of non-response to CC is significantly increased in patients who are obese, insulin resistant or hyperandrogenic compared with those who respond. Therefore, initial screening parameters before CC administration are required in order to identify patients at risk of remaining anovulatory. Predictive factors for a poor prognosis of ovulation are: increased free androgen index, obesity, increased ovarian volume and amenorrhea[13]. In addition, at least in Japanese women, 120-minute levels of blood glucose and blood glucose × insulin after a 75-g fasting glucose load seem to be other valid biochemical markers of CC resistance[14].

In addition, pharmacogenetic variability in metabolism of the drug may account for the lack of response. Indeed, it has been suggested that variability in the metabolism of zyclomiphene influences its dosage requirement. Therefore, monitoring plasma drug concentration might enable the response to CC to be predicted in individual patients at an early stage of their treatment, thereby increasing the benefit/cost ratio of treatment[3].

Failure to conceive (CC failure)

The usual discrepancy between ovulation and pregnancy rates (about 50% of those who ovulate will conceive) can be explained by several factors.

First, the peripheral antiestrogenic effect of CC at the level of the cervical mucus and endometrium is presumably important. The alteration of cervical mucus attested by a negative post-coital test may be overcome by performing IUI. In contrast, the constant suppression of endometrial proliferation attested by ultrasound at the time of ovulation, which seems to be unrelated to the dose and duration of treatment, justifies recommending alternative therapies.

Second, increased LH secretion which results from the hypothalamic effect of CC is likely to compromise pregnancy rate with an increased risk of miscarriage. However, the mechanism whereby increased LH exerts a deleterious effect is unknown.

Finally, age and amenorrhea have also been reported as being relevant predictors for live birth after CC treatment[11,13].

A course of six treatment cycles with CC is usually recommended in WHO group II anovulatory women. Nevertheless, 71–87.5% of pregnancies achieved with CC occur within the first three cycles of treatment[9,13]. In properly selected candidates, the cumulative pregnancy rate may reach 60% after six cycles[10]. The failure to conceive within a maximum of six CC-induced cycles with proven ovulation is a clear indication for expanding the diagnostic evaluation to exclude other infertility factors or for changing the overall treatment strategy if evaluation is already complete.

ADJUVANT THERAPIES

Insulin sensitizers

Insulin secretion should be carefully assessed in women with WHO group II anovulation. Indeed, insulin interferes with the process of folliculogenesis

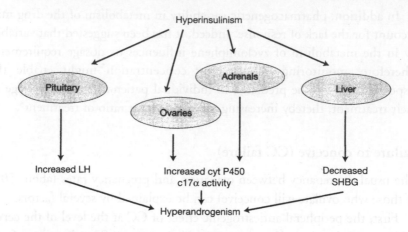

Figure 5.2 Effects of insulin on androgen production

by acting at the pituitary, ovarian and hepatic levels (Figure 5.2). *In vitro* studies have demonstrated the ability of insulin to release pituitary LH and to increase the stimulatory effects of LH on theca cell androgen production through stimulation of cytochrome P450 c17α. Furthermore, insulin reduces the hepatic production of sex hormone binding globulin (SHBG), a protein involved in the binding of steroids, which results in higher serum concentrations of active free androgens. Thus, insulin hypersecretion is likely to contribute to the process of anovulation by modifying the androgenic environment.

Therefore, it is of prime importance, at the initial clinical set-up, to detect a state of insulin resistance responsible for hyperinsulinemia and hyperandrogenemia. Major determinants of insulin resistance are central obesity, body mass index (BMI) and PCOS. However, insulin resistance is also reported in lean women with PCOS.

Weight loss and lifestyle modifications are the first-line therapy in obese anovulatory women. Indeed, resumption of regular menses and spontaneous ovulation can be observed after even a slight weight reduction. It has been shown that a weight loss of 5% compared with basal level can significantly increase the ovulation rate in anovulatory obese patients. However, the majority of patients are not able to lose weight without medical treatment and, consequently, physicians are encouraged to use insulin-lowering drugs.

Metformin is an insulin sensitizer currently prescribed in patients with type 2 diabetes for its ability to improve insulin sensitivity and to reduce insulin secretion. Thus, this drug is indirectly able to lower clinical and chemical hyperandrogenism. An additional direct effect of metformin on ovarian theca cells, demonstrated *in vitro*[15,16], is likely to participate in the reduction of androgen secretion. While metformin may be effective *per se* to restore ovulation, the issue to be addressed in this part of the chapter is related to its ability to improve the effectiveness of CC therapy. It should be kept in mind that both obesity and hyperandrogenemia have been described as negative predictive factors for ovulation rate in CC-treated patients. Therefore, the rationale to add metformin derives from the potential benefit of this adjuvant therapy to improve the effectiveness of CC. Two meta-analyses have recently shown that metformin + CC is more effective than CC alone in achieving ovulation and pregnancy[17,18]. However, these meta-analyses were performed on the basis of studies with a small number of patients. Moreover, other recent large randomized controlled trials comparing CC alone and CC + metformin could not demonstrate any significant differences. Finally, it is still unclear whether metformin should be prescribed only in patients with insulin resistance, as its effectiveness in restoring ovulation in non-obese, non-insulin-resistant anovulatory patients has also been demonstrated. Additional trials are required to define which patients could benefit from this adjuvant therapy.

Dexamethasone

In some CC-resistant patients, mostly in hyperandrogenic women with PCOS and elevated levels of dehydroepiandrosterone (DHEAS), addition of dexamethazone at a dose of 0.5 mg in the evening may induce ovulation when CC alone has failed. However, glucocorticoid treatment stimulates appetite and weight gain and should be reserved for women with late-onset 21-hydroxylase deficiency.

Human chorionic gonadotropin

The use of human chorionic gonadotropin (hCG) to trigger ovulation is difficult to justify on a routine basis because spontaneous ovulation is likely to occur. Even in CC-treated patients undergoing IUI, there is no evidence that hCG administration is more effective than detection of the endogenous LH surge. Therefore, use of exogenous hCG could be limited to those women who require IUI and in whom a midcycle LH surge cannot reliably be detected[19].

SIDE-EFFECTS OF CC

Vasomotor flushes occur in approximately 10% of CC-treated women during CC intake. Mood swings are also common. Visual disturbances, including blurred or double vision, scotomas and light sensitivity are observed in < 2% of women and are reversible.

The main side-effects are linked to the antiestrogenic effects of CC on peripheral target tissues. The quality and quantity of cervical mucus production is sometimes reduced and the ability of spermatozoa to cross the cervical barrier may be diminished. Furthermore, endometrial thickness may be either reduced or heterogeneous at the time of hCG administration and could explain the discrepancy observed between ovulation and pregnancy rates.

In those cases with reduced endometrial thickness, tamoxifen has been suggested as an alternative to CC. This non-steroidal selective estrogen receptor modulator (SERM) acts as an agonist on cervical mucus and endometrium. However, a recent meta-analysis of four studies comparing the two treatments and including 921 cycles (273 women) could not demonstrate any benefit of tamoxifen over CC as regards ovulation (OR 0.755, 95% CI 0.513, 1.111), pregnancy per cycle (OR 1.056, 95% CI 0.583, 1.912) or per ovulatory cycle (OR 1.162, 95% CI 0.632, 2.134)[20]. While none of the trials was powered or designed to detect differences in side-effects, tamoxifen may be an option in women suffering from intolerable side-effects of CC. However, patients may have concerns about taking a medication commonly used as chemotherapy for breast cancer. Overall, the familiarity of clinicians with the dosing regimens and side-effects of CC makes this therapeutic agent more suitable for clinical use compared with tamoxifen.

Finally, a recent analysis of eight case–control studies concluded that neither fertility drug use nor use for more than 12 months was associated with invasive ovarian cancer[21]. However, prolonged treatment with CC is generally futile and should be avoided[19].

INDICATION IN NORMO-OVULATORY WOMEN

CC has been proposed for ovarian stimulation in normo-ovulatory women with unexplained infertility and/or for women undergoing IUI treatment. The rationale behind this is that CC overcomes subtle defects in ovarian function and/or increases the number of preovulatory follicles. The success rate was notably lower than in anovulatory women[22]. A recent meta-analysis of six randomized clinical trials[23] has reported that CC appeared to be superior to no treatment or placebo. Indeed, the common odds ratios for clinical pregnancy per patient and per treatment cycle were 2.37 (1.22–4.62) and 2.5 (1.35–4.62), respectively. The authors concluded that, given the easy use, low cost and low incidence of side-effects, CC should be considered as a primary treatment for persistent unexplained infertility. However, as discussed later in another section of this book, the effectiveness of CC therapy is clearly lower than that observed with the use of gonadotropin preparations.

CONCLUSIONS

While it has been more than 40 years since CC was first introduced into clinical practice, this medication remains the first-line therapy for women with ovulatory dysfunction. This is because it is a cheap, easy to use therapy and has an acceptable efficiency. However, as discussed in other chapters low-dose gonadotropin treatment, as well as administration of aromatase inhibitors, may replace CC as first-line treatment in the future.

5.2 Gonadotropins

INTRODUCTION

Gonadotropins are extensively used in patients suffering from chronic anovulation. According to the World Health Organization (WHO) classification, impairments of ovarian function can be separated into different groups:

- WHO group I: characterized by a profound deficiency of both endogenous follicle stimulating hormone (FSH) and luteinizing hormone (LH) secretion attested by amenorrhea, related to functional or organic hypothalamic disorders

- WHO group II: so-called 'normogonadotropic anovulation' separated into two subgroups – WHO IIa characterized by a qualitative disorder of the pulsatile gonadotropin secretion and WHO IIb, a primary ovarian dysfunction (polycystic ovaries) where the inadequate gonadotropin secretion results from the acyclic ovarian production of steroids

- WHO group III: characterized by the inability of the ovaries to respond to FSH (ovarian failure)

WHO group II anovulation, including PCOS, is a common disease for women of reproductive age. Gonadotropins are currently recommended as a second-line therapy when CC has failed. However, this strategy has recently been challenged.

Apart from these anovulatory disorders, gonadotropins are frequently prescribed for inducing a mild stimulation in normo-ovulatory women enrolled in an ovulation induction (OI)/intrauterine insemination (IUI) program. Therefore, ovarian stimulation by gonadotropins plays a central role in modern infertility treatment.

During the past decades, one major advance in the management of chronic anovulation arose from the application of physiological concepts for folliculogenesis. Indeed, a better knowledge of the respective roles of FSH and LH in single dominant follicle selection has led to the development of novel ovulation induction regimens for anovulatory women. These have significantly enhanced the efficacy of gonadotropin treatment while reducing the risk of complications such as high-order multiple pregnancies. Moreover, successive advances in the manufacturing process have allowed improvements to be made in the purity and consistency of the products and enabled consistent recombinant FSH as well as LH and human chorionic gonadotropin (hCG) preparations to be produced. Application of recombinant technologies to gonadotropin production has largely contributed to the increase of both safety and efficacy of ovarian stimulation regimens.

STRUCTURE

FSH, LH and hCG are three gonadotropins currently used in clinical practice for stimulation of follicular development and ovulation induction. These molecules belong to a family of glycoproteins which share structural similarities. They are heterodimers, containing two non-covalently linked proteins, named α and β subunits. These subunits are encoded by separate genes. Within an animal species, the amino acid sequences of the α subunits of all gonadotropins are identical, whereas the β subunits differ and confer biological specificity on the individual gonadotropins. Both α and β subunits are glycosylated. As shown in Figure 5.3, the α and β subunits of FSH and LH have asparagine (N)-linked glycosylation sites, while the C-terminal β chain of hCG has additional serine (O)-linked sites. Glycosylation is a very complex step that takes place in the endoplasmic reticulum. The final structure of the Asn-linked carbohydrates differs between gonadotropins. In FSH and hCG the terminal residues on the carbohydrate antenna consist of sialic acid while LH carbohydrates terminate with sulfate-4-N-acetyl-galactosamine.

The carbohydrates on the gonadotropins serve many important functions. They are required for proper three-dimensional structure of the molecules and for binding to their corresponding receptors. Therefore, carbohydrates are highly relevant to biological activity. It is well established that

121

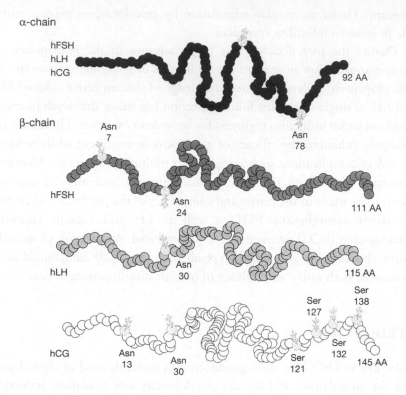

α-chain

hFSH
hLH
hCG

92 AA

β-chain   Asn
                  7
                              Asn
                               78

hFSH
          Asn
           24   111 AA

Asn
 30   115 AA

                              Ser
                         Ser   138
                         127

                                    Ser
hCG   Asn   Ser   132
           13   Asn   121   145 AA
                  30

Figure 5.3 Schematic representation of the primary structure of α and β subunits of the gonadotropin family. Glycosylation sites in each subunit are indicated. Reproduced with permission from Olijve W, *et al*. Mol Hum Reprod 1996; 2: 371–82

glycosylation determines the half-life of gonadotropins. The increased *in vivo* bioactivity and longer plasma half-life of hCG compared with those of LH are attributed to the four additional O-linked oligosaccharides on the C-terminal peptide.

In conclusion, glycosylation is an absolute requirement for full biological activity of the glycoprotein hormones.

FSH displays extensive microheterogeneity which is reflected in different individual FSH isoforms. This is a result of different types of carbohydrate chain combinations and different degrees of terminal sialylation (Figure 5.4) Differences in the degree of sialylation result in basic–acidic charge differences. This provides the basis for differences in receptor binding activity, biological activity and metabolic clearance rate. On the basis of differences in isoelectric points, investigators have shown that human pituitary FSH can be separated into at least 20 isoform fractions. More acidic isoforms (high

122

sialic acid content) have been shown to exhibit reduced receptor binding affinity and *in vitro* bioactivity, whereas circulating half-life and, therefore, *in vivo* bioactivity assessed by the Steelman–Pohley assay are extended[24]. However, results may differ from one bioassay to another and *in vitro* assessment does not correlate with *in vivo* FSH bioactivity.

PRODUCTION

FSH and LH preparations

Over the past 40 years, gonadotropins have been used extensively in the treatment of female infertility. During the first three decades, only human urine-derived gonadotropin preparations were available, or human pituitary extracts were used. Recent advances in biotechnology have led to the development of recombinant preparations.

Urine-derived preparations

Early preparations containing FSH and LH were obtained by extraction and concentration of minute amounts of gonadotropins from the urine of postmenopausal women. The end result was a rather crude preparation of human menopausal gonadotropin (hMG) with a low specific activity. In addition, because of its impurity, allergic reactions were occasionally reported.

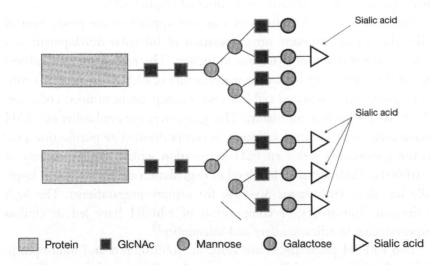

Figure 5.4 Sialic acid content determines the different isoforms of the FSH molecule

As FSH is the most important hormone required for folliculogenesis, the need for an improved product, combined with advances in purification techniques, led to u-hFSH, which contained mainly FSH activity with little LH contamination. Although u-hFSH had improved specific activity compared with hMG, 95% of the proteins present were non-gonadotropic substances. Then, highly purified u-hFSH, a preparation containing more than 95% pure FSH, with a specific activity of more than 9000 IU FSH/mg, came close to the 'ideal FSH'.

Both u-hFSH and highly purified u-hFSH showed improvements in pregnancy rates compared with hMG. However, these preparations still had inherent disadvantages: all urine-derived preparations required the collection of vast quantities of urine (a poor-quality starting material), leading to unreliable supply and, most importantly, batch-to-batch inconsistency. Therefore, replacement of these urinary preparations was initiated in the early 1990s.

Development of recombinant preparations

Although the recombinant production of simple proteins is increasingly common, gonadotropin hormones represented a particular challenge. Early recombinant DNA products were expressed in bacterial cells but these cells are incapable of carrying out post-translational modifications, such as glycosylation. As gonadotropins require glycosylation for full biological activity, recombinant gonadotropins were produced by genetically engineered mammalian cells (Chinese hamster ovary (CHO) cells), into which the genes encoding the α and β subunits were inserted (Figure 5.5).

Recombinant DNA technology was first applied to the production of FSH, the crucial hormone for stimulation of follicular development and thus for management of ovulation induction. The most significant advantage of this technology is that the manufacture of r-hFSH starts with a constant genetically engineered cell line and is independent of urine collection which has an inconsistent quality. This guarantees the availability of a FSH preparation, with minimal variation in composition. The purification procedure consistently yields an FSH preparation with a specific activity of > 10 000 IU FSH/mg and a low level of degradation and/or oxidation (typically less than 10% versus 30–40% for urinary preparations). The high purity and consistency of composition of r-hFSH have led to clinical improvements in efficacy, safety and tolerability[25].

Two r-hFSH preparations are available: follitropin-α and follitropin-β. Although similar recombinant techniques have been used for transfecting

124

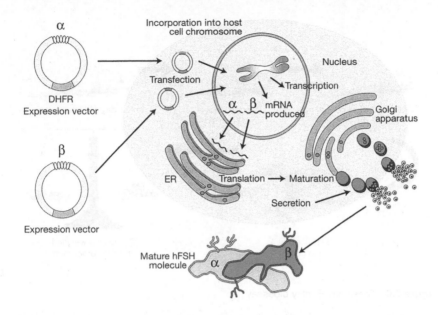

Figure 5.5 Expression of recombinant human follicle stimulating hormone in Chinese hamster ovary cells. Reproduced with permission from Howles CM. *Hum Reprod Update* 1996; 2: 172–91

mammalian cell lines with the human FSH genes, commercial manufacturing and purification are slightly different.

Despite the complexity of post-translational modification, the isoform distribution of r-hFSH produced in a CHO cell line and grown in perfusion culture is similar to that observed with pituitary FSH and u-hFSH, although r-hFSH contains slightly more basic isoforms than u-hFSH, despite structural and biochemical similarity.

In the late 1990s, another step forward came with the 'filled by mass' procedure. Indeed, while the manufacturing process of recombinant preparations was highly controlled, the final step, the calibration process, was still dependent on the rat Steelman–Pohley bioassay (Figure 5.6). It consists of measurement of the ovarian weight after once daily injections of FSH for 3 days to prepubertal rats. The major drawback of this bioassay is related to the huge variability usually observed with the results based on this assay (ovarian weight measurement). For that reason, according to the European Pharmacopeia regulation, a large range (80–125%) in the declared content of gonadotropins based on the bioassay is accepted. This means that, in one ampule labeled as 75 IU FSH, the actual FSH content may vary between 60

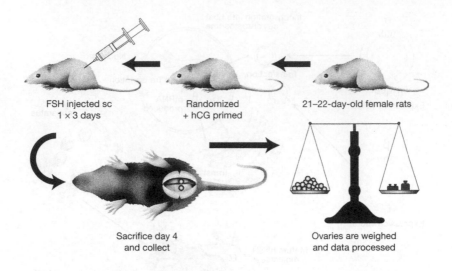

Figure 5.6 Steelman–Pohley bioassay

and 92 IU or even more, owing to the fact that the values 80% and 125% are not absolute but also have a range.

This huge range in the potency estimation of the final product can explain the intraindividual variability that has been reported from one cycle to another with the use of preparations released according to the Steelman–Pohley bioassay. This issue is critical because the choice of starting dose is a major determining factor to prevent the risk of overstimulation or cancellation in the management of ovarian stimulation.

Owing to improvements in the manufacturing process of recombinant follitropin-α it became possible to produce batches of recombinant follitropin-α with an almost identical FSH-isoform profile. As the isoform profile clearly determines the FSH bioactivity this made it possible to fill recombinant follitropin-α by mass which is measured by an accurate size-exclusion high pressure liquid chromatography (SE-HPLC) method (Figure 5.7).

The main advantage of this method compared with the Steelman–Pohley bioassay is that its variability for measuring the FSH content is less than 2% compared with approximately 20% variability with the Steelman–Pohley assay. This procedure was applied for the first time to follitropin-α in the late 1990s. Follitropin-α produced through recombinant technology has a high specific bioactivity (13.750 IU/mg). The equivalent of 75 IU FSH

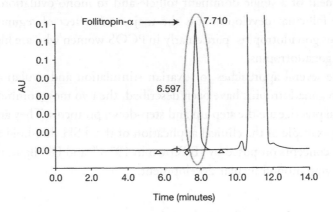

Figure 5.7 Identification of follitropin-α as a single peak with HPLC allowing its measure in mass

filled by the bioassay is 5.5 μg r-hFSH filled by mass. As discussed later in this section, the filled-by-mass process has significantly improved the consistency of the ovarian response to FSH, reduced the need for dose adjustment and reduced the risk of cancellation caused by low or over-response.

Similar technology has been applied to produce r-hLH and r-hCG preparations which have been brought onto the market recently. These recombinant products have pharmacodynamic and pharmacokinetic properties comparable with those of native hormones. In addition, they are also extremely pure and consistent from batch to batch. They are also measured by mass (micrograms) and are currently used in clinical practice.

These significant improvements of the manufacturing and calibration processes of gonadotropin production have provided new tools for clinicians to conduct the protocols for ovarian stimulation properly. Moreover, each preparation can be prescribed separately in order to adjust hormonal supply to each woman's characteristics and according to the stage of follicular development. These advances have allowed us to mimic more accurately the endocrine events that occur in the physiological cycle.

PROTOCOLS FOR CHRONIC ANOVULATION

The main objective of ovulation induction in women with chronic anovulation is to stimulate with a hormonal sequence which will lead to the development of a single dominant follicle and to mono-ovulation. Indeed, multiple follicular development is the major side-effect of regimens using exogenous gonadotropins, particularly in PCOS women who are highly sensitive to gonadotropins.

While several approaches for ovarian stimulation and ovulation induction with gonadotropins have been described, the two most commonly used in clinical practice are the step-up and step-down protocols. They are an outstanding example of the clinical application of the 'FSH threshold and FSH window' concepts proposed by JB Brown in 1978[26] and DT Baird in 1987[27] for achieving monofollicular development.

FSH therapy: lessons from physiology

The later stages of follicle maturation, from antrum formation to ovulation, are regulated by the cyclical changes in LH and FSH secretion. Increased FSH concentration, which occurs during the luteofollicular transition, is a potent stimulus for follicular recruitment and several early antral follicles start to enlarge beyond 2–5 mm. Subsequent development of this cohort during the follicular phase becomes dependent on sustained stimulation by gonadotropins[28]. Each growing follicle has a specific threshold level for FSH

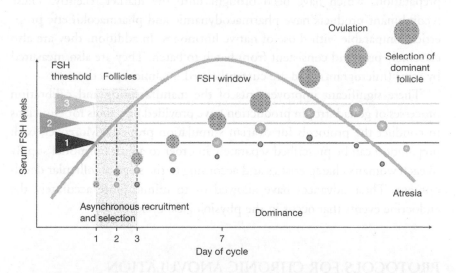

Figure 5.8 FSH-dependent events during the follicular phase. This schematic shows that three follicles with different FSH thresholds are recruited during the early follicular phase. The leading follicle which has the lowest FSH threshold is preserved from atresia in the late follicular phase when serum FSH declines

that should be surpassed to ensure ongoing development[26] (Figure 5.8). This concept of 'FSH threshold' led to the recommendation of a stepwise FSH increment during ovarian stimulation in order to recruit a limited number of the more FSH-sensitive follicles.

During the late follicular phase, FSH concentrations decline in response to the negative feedback exerted at the pituitary level by increasing levels of estradiol and inhibin B. The first recruited follicle (selected follicle), which is highly sensitive to FSH, continues its growth, whereas fewer FSH-sensitive follicles are driven to atresia. This concept of 'FSH window' means that, as long as FSH concentration is above the threshold, follicular growth will continue. The duration of this 'FSH window' during which FSH concentrations are above the threshold required to stimulate ongoing development determines the number of follicles that can develop to the pre-ovulatory stage[27,29]. Application of this concept of the FSH window was described as the step-down protocol.

STEP-UP PROTOCOLS

Conventional and low-dose protocols

According to this protocol, daily starting doses of 75 IU FSH treatment may be increased by 75 IU FSH every 5–7 days if no selected follicle (10 mm in diameter) is apparent on ultrasound (Figure 5.9). While an ovulation rate of 70% is achieved, the incidence of multiple pregnancy was unacceptable (36% of pregnancies) as well as the frequency of potentially life-threatening ovarian hyperstimulation syndrome (OHSS) (14%). Therefore, it has been stated that the conventional protocol should not be employed to induce ovulation in patients with WHO group II anovulation. A similar conclusion was drawn if the dose adjustment was performed after 7 days but was reduced to half of the starting dose (low-dose protocol). It was concluded that the duration of the initial starting dose is essential to prevent the risk of overstimulation.

Chronic low-dose protocols

In order to minimize the risk of multifollicular development, a 'softer' regimen, the so-called 'chronic low-dose step-up' protocol, has been proposed. This regimen stipulates that a starting dose of 75 IU/day should be

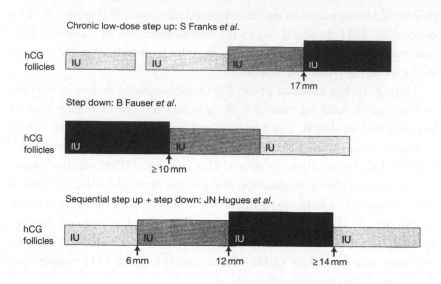

Figure 5.9 Schematic representation of the three forms of step protocols[29,36,37]

maintained for up to 14 days (Figure 5.9). If no ovarian response is noted after 14 days, the daily FSH dose is increased by 37.5 IU. Any further FSH increment thereafter is made by 37.5 IU at weekly intervals to a maximum of 225 IU/day. When the first recruited follicle emerges with a diameter of ≥ 10 mm, the dose of FSH (the threshold dose for the most sensitive follicle) is maintained until the follicle reaches a mean diameter of 17 mm. At that point, hCG at a dose of 250 µg is administered. If there are more than three follicles of 15 mm or greater in diameter, the cycle is canceled due to the risk of multiple pregnancy and/or OHSS. If there is no follicular response after 35 days of treatment, the cycle is canceled. When, despite ovulation, pregnancy has not occurred during the first course of treatment, FSH is reintroduced at a subthreshold dose (37.5 IU less than the preceding threshold dose). In women who develop multiple follicles using the above-mentioned protocol, the treatment is modified so that a smaller starting dose (37.5 IU) is used and/or the chosen increments are lower than usual.

Conventional and chronic low-dose step-up protocols yield comparable pregnancy rates[30,31]. However, the major advantage of the chronic low-dose step-up protocol is the high rate of monofollicular development which is about 69% (54–88%)[32]. The reported fecundity per cycle is around 20% (12–45%); the multiple pregnancy rate is about 6% and the incidence of OHSS is 0.14% (0–2.4%)[33].

The rationale to keep the same FSH dosage when the selected follicle is apparent is related to the integrity of the hypothalamic–pituitary–ovarian axis. Consequently, endogenous FSH concentrations actually decrease during the final part of the ovarian stimulation. This leads to closure of the FSH window which is essential to avoid multifollicular development[34]. Thus, concomitant use of gonadotropin releasing hormone analogs (GnRH-a), which will block the feedback at the pituitary level, is not recommended. Indeed, a recent Cochrane Library meta-analysis reported a higher overstimulation rate when a GnRH-a was added to gonadotropin treatment (odds ratio 3.15; 95% CI 1.48, 6.70)[35].

As regards the starting dose of FSH, 75 IU has traditionally been used but this obviously needs to be adjusted according to several parameters such as body mass index (BMI), patient characteristics (particularly PCOS appearance at ultrasound) and the history of previous response to FSH therapy. In patients with PCOS, Franks et al.[36] concluded from a large series that a starting dose of 52.5 IU for 14 days was appropriate. Indeed, a retrospective comparison of the two starting doses (75 IU versus 52.5 IU) has shown that the rate of monofollicular development was higher with the lower starting dose (72 vs. 84%). The rates of ovulation, pregnancy and miscarriage were similar. In highly FSH-sensitive patients, Balasch et al.[38] have shown that starting doses of 50 IU and 37.5 IU of rFSH, with dose increments by 25 IU and 18.5 IU, respectively, may be required. In those patients, similar monofollicular development rates can be achieved. These authors concluded that even a starting dose of 37.5 IU of rFSH may be sufficient to induce follicular growth.

It is believed that strict adherence to a 14-day starting period using a persistent dose is essential to minimize the risk of multifollicular development. Indeed, Homburg and Howles[33] have compared cycle outcomes when a starting FSH dose of 75 IU was administered for 14 or 7 days before any incremental dose of 37.5 IU if necessary. While the 7-day starting regimen allowed a significant decrease in the amount of FSH required (mean 17.1 vs. 22.1 ampules) and a decreased mean duration of treatment (13.1 vs. 17.4 days), there was no difference in the daily effective dose, number of canceled cycles, estradiol concentrations and number of large and intermediate follicles. Moreover, pregnancy rates for the 7-day and 14-day protocols were similar (56 and 40% per patient and 33 and 19% per completed cycle, respectively). However, the 7-day protocol led to a multiple pregnancy rate of 24% compared with 0% in the 14-day protocol. Therefore, it seems essential to maintain the initial dose for 14 days before increasing the daily FSH dose.

In addition, the multiple pregnancy rate can be reduced by strict application of criteria for administering hCG. In that respect, hCG must be withheld in the presence of more than three follicles of >15 mm in diameter. Indeed, as reported from the Serono database[39], the pregnancy rates were 17, 26, 34 and 26% when 1, 2, 3 and >3 follicles exceeding 15 mm in diameter were present on the day of hCG administration. However, the multiple birth rate increased dramatically, the respective figures being 5, 12, 20 and 50%.

Overall data collected with the chronic low-dose regimen indicate that this protocol is effective and safe. White et al.[36] reported the cumulative conception rate as 57% after six cycles; 75% of pregnancies occurred in the first three cycles of treatment and only one pregnancy occurred after the sixth cycle.

Step-down protocol

In an attempt to mimic physiology more closely, a stimulation regimen has been described by Fauser's group for women with PCOS. This regimen proposes to start stimulation with a loading dose of FSH (150 IU) which allows the threshold of the most FSH-sensitive follicles to be surpassed (Figure 5.9). Thereafter, in accordance with the concept of the FSH window, the daily FSH dose is reduced in a stepwise fashion (112.5 and 75 IU every 3 days) as soon as follicles of ≥10 mm have emerged from the cohort[40,41]. Monitoring of a step-down cycle needs more experience compared with a low-dose step-up regimen for two reasons. First, an inadequate loading dose exposes the patient to the risk of uncontrolled multifollicular recruitment. Second, a premature reduction of FSH doses may induce atresia of the whole cohort.

COMPARISON OF STEP-UP AND STEP-DOWN PROTOCOLS

Few studies have compared both effectiveness and safety of the chronic low-dose step-up and step-down protocols. Van Santbrink and Fauser[41], in a small prospective randomized controlled trial (37 clomiphene citrate-resistant women), reported comparable clinical outcomes but a substantially reduced stimulation period (9 days vs. 18 days). In addition, a higher rate of monofollicular cycles (88 vs. 56%) was observed in the step-down group. Balasch et al.[42], using a crossover study design, compared the low-dose step-up protocol with a modified step-down protocol with 300 IU of r-hFSH on cycle day 3, no treatment on the next 3 days (cycle days 4–6) and 75 IU r-hFSH on cycle day 7 until cycle day 9). These authors concluded that the step-down approach appears to be more physiological because it reduces the risk of multifollicular development. However, in a recent large multicenter study[43], the step-up protocol using r-hFSH appeared more efficient in obtaining monofollicular development (68.2 vs. 32%; $p < 0.0001$) than the step-down protocol. Furthermore, a higher rate of multifollicular development (36 vs. 4.7%; $p < 0.0001$) and a higher cancellation rate (38 vs. 15%; $p < 0.001$) were observed in the step-down compared with the step-up group. There was an increase in hyperstimulation in the step-down group (11 vs. 2.25%; $p < 0.001$).

Several differences may account for the conflicting results between these studies. PCOS is a heterogeneous disorder and patients' characteristics were different with a 'milder' form of PCOS (normal mean BMI, lower hyperandrogenism) in the study by Christin-Maitre and Hugues[43]. It is likely that a lower starting dose (100 IU) for a subset of patients with PCOS might have reduced the risk of overstimulation in the step-down group. These findings underline the need for optimization of the starting doses for both step-up and step-down protocols. Such optimization should prevent hyperstimulation due to a starting dose far above the FSH threshold or should minimize the time-consuming low-dose increments by starting with a higher dose in women with an augmented FSH threshold.

As recommended by Fauser's group[41], the strategy could be to start with a chronic low-dose step-up regimen in order to determine the individual FSH threshold dose. Thereafter, a step-down regimen could be applied with a starting dose of 37.5 IU above the FSH threshold dose.

SEQUENTIAL STEP-UP AND STEP-DOWN PROTOCOL

Applying the two concepts of FSH threshold and FSH window, Hugues et al.[37] developed the so-called 'sequential step-up and step-down protocol' (Figure 5.9). Following a low-dose step-up regimen, the FSH dose is reduced by half when the leading follicle reaches a diameter of 14 mm. In a prospective randomized controlled trial, these authors observed that cycles treated with the sequential protocol exhibited significantly lower estradiol concentrations and a lower number of medium-sized (14–15 mm) follicles. They concluded that decreasing the FSH dose following the step-up follicular selection might be an effective tool to reduce the risk of multifollicular development.

PREDICTIVE FACTORS FOR OVULATION AND PREGNANCY

The importance of the initial patient screening has recently been highlighted in order to help in the choice of FSH starting dose, to prevent the risk of multifollicular development and to predict the chance of ongoing pregnancy. Fauser's group in Rotterdam largely contributed to defining the most relevant factors.

Prediction of the threshold FSH dose is essential for optimizing cycle outcome using step protocols. The BMI is an important prognostic factor that influences the FSH threshold and the cycle cancellation rate due to absence of ovarian response. Furthermore, Imani *et al.*[44] established a model for prediction of the FSH threshold using multivariate analysis in order to increase the safety and efficiency of low-dose protocols. Significant predictors for the FSH response dose were defined: BMI, presence of CC

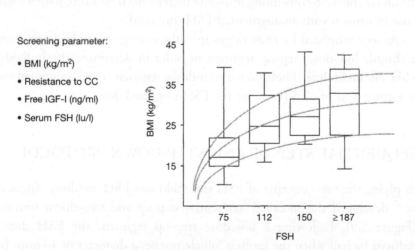

Figure 5.10 Predictive factors for the FSH response in normogonadotropic anovulatory women treated with a chronic low-dose protocol

resistance, initial free insulin-like growth factor-I and initial serum FSH concentrations were positively correlated with the FSH dose required to attain the threshold (Figure 5.10).

In addition, chances for multiple follicular development during FSH induction of ovulation have also been assessed in normogonadotropic anovulatory women treated with a step-up protocol for the first cycle and a step-down regimen for all subsequent cycles[45]. Chances for multifollicular development could be predicted by initial hyperandrogenism (androstenedione, testosterone), raised LH concentrations as well as by increased antral follicle count (polycystic ovaries). In addition, chances for ongoing pregnancy can be predicted on the basis of age of the woman, testosterone and IGF-I concentrations.

A meta-analysis of 13 studies recently reported patient predictive factors for outcome of gonadotropin stimulation in women with normogonadotropic anovulatory infertility[46]. Significant associations were found for the total amount of FSH administered, cancellation rate, ovulation rate and miscarriage rate with BMI. Furthermore, significant associations were found for the total amount of FSH and pregnancy rate with insulin resistance. The authors concluded that the most clinically useful predictors for the outcome of gonadotropin stimulation in normogonadotropic women are obesity and insulin resistance.

TYPE OF GONADOTROPINS

From a theoretical point of view, the choice of gonadotropins (exogenous FSH ± LH) should be made according to the specific disorder responsible for the anovulatory process. It is well established that both exogenous FSH and LH are required in women suffering from WHO group I anovulation. In contrast, administration of FSH alone should be sufficient in the other forms of anovulation where baseline LH secretion is maintained or even increased. However, in clinical practice, the ongoing controversy about the type of gonadotropin preparations that should be used is mainly related to cost-effectiveness issues.

Furthermore, it has been widely demonstrated that the success of ovarian stimulation depends more on the type of regimen, with strict adherence to a low-dose stepwise protocol, rather than on the presence or absence of LH in the preparations.

Nevertheless, the improvement in the manufacturing process of gonadotropins during the past decades led to a comparison of the effectiveness and safety of different preparations. The vast majority of clinical studies have been performed in patients with anovulation related to PCOS. However, the definition of PCOS was quite heterogeneous and any comparison between studies should take into account overall confounding factors usually observed in the selection of patients. Moreover, in most of the analyses, the authors indicated that the methodological quality of the trials was fairly poor and that tentative conclusions must be interpreted with caution.

u-hMG versus u-hFSH

The first meta-analysis on the comparison between u-hMG and u-hFSH was conducted in 1996 and was based on six randomized studies performed between 1985 and 1991[47]. No significant difference could be demonstrated between u-hFSH and hMG in terms of pregnancy rate. However, potential advantages in terms of purity and a possible reduction in OHSS risk led the authors to recommend the use of FSH preparations.

In a larger Cochrane Library meta-analysis, the effectiveness of u-hMG and u-hFSH for ovarian stimulation was compared in 14 randomized trials[35]. Gonadotropin protocols in the included studies were quite heterogeneous (low-dose step-up or conventional protocols with concomitant GnRH-a administration in four trials). No significant differences were demonstrated in cycle outcomes, except for a reduction in the risk of OHSS (OR 0.33; 95% CI 0.16, 0.65) when u-hFSH was used. Moreover, the beneficial effect of u-hFSH versus u-hMG for OHSS (6 vs. 12%) was observed only when GnRH-a was not administered concomitantly (OR 0.20; 95% CI 0.08, 0.46).

These data allow the following conclusions to be drawn:

(1) The use of FSH preparations should be recommended for the subgroup of PCOS patients to reduce the risk of OHSS.

(2) There is no advantage in using GnRH-a, which do not prevent the risk of overstimulation and increase the overall cost of stimulation. These data indirectly confirmed that LH hypersecretion is not the main factor responsible in the pathogenesis of anovulation in PCOS patients.

u-hFSH versus r-hFSH

In several randomized controlled trials comparing the efficiency of low-dose step-up regimens with u-hFSH and r-hFSH administration, a higher incidence of monofollicular development was observed in the r-hFSH group. Moreover, the mean daily FSH dose required to achieve the threshold of follicular selection has been reported to be lower when using r-hFSH compared with u-hFSH[48]. These data support previous *in vitro* reports revealing a higher biopotency of recombinant preparations.

With regards to the safety and effectiveness of u-hFSH and r-hFSH, a recent Cochrane Library meta-analysis of randomized controlled trials was performed in PCOS women[49]. All trials used a chronic low-dose scheme. In two of them, a significant reduction in the duration of stimulation and in the total dose could be demonstrated. However, there was no significant difference regarding ovulation rate (OR 1.19; 95% CI 0.78, 1.80), pregnancy rate (OR 0.95; 95% CI 0.64, 1.41), miscarriage rate (OR 1.26; 95% CI 0.59, 2.70), multiple pregnancy rate (OR 0.44; 95% CI 0.16, 1.21) and OHSS (OR 1.55; 95% CI 0.50, 4.84) (Figure 5.11). Therefore, there is as yet insufficient evidence to conclude that r-hFSH is more effective than u-hFSH for ovulation in women with CC-resistant PCOS. If the use of r-hFSH leads to a lower dosage requirement and shorter stimulation period, it is still questionable whether r-hFSH is also more cost-effective, because r-hFSH preparations are more expensive than u-hFSH.

Preparations filled by bioassay versus those filled by mass

Due to the relatively recent availability of the 'filled-by-mass' preparations, few studies have been reported so far to assess the benefit of this new calibration process. A large prospective multicenter study comparing the respective efficacy and safety of follitropin-α filled by mass and filled by bioassay was performed in women with normogonadotropic anovulation treated for three cycles according to a chronic low-dose step-up protocol[50]. The authors showed that the number of treatment days, the need for FSH dose adjustment as well as the number of canceled cycles were significantly reduced with the use of preparations filled by mass. These results reveal a higher batch-to-batch consistency of these new products. As a consequence, cost-effectiveness has been much improved.

Outcome	rFSH (n/N)	uFSH (n/N)		OR (95% CI)
Ovulation per cycle	182/255	142/202		1.19 (0.78–1.80)
Clinical pregnancy per cycle	306/934	251/882		0.95 (0.64–1.41)
Ongoing pregnancy per woman	68/611	139/603		1.10 (0.51–2.35)
Miscarriage per woman	168/546	139/533		1.22 (0.60–2.46)
OHSS per woman	22/189	19/158		1.59 (0.50–4.84)
Multiple pregnancy per woman	5/231	12/86		0.44 (0.16–1.19)
Cancellation rate	42/223	24/138		1.10 (0.64–1.91)

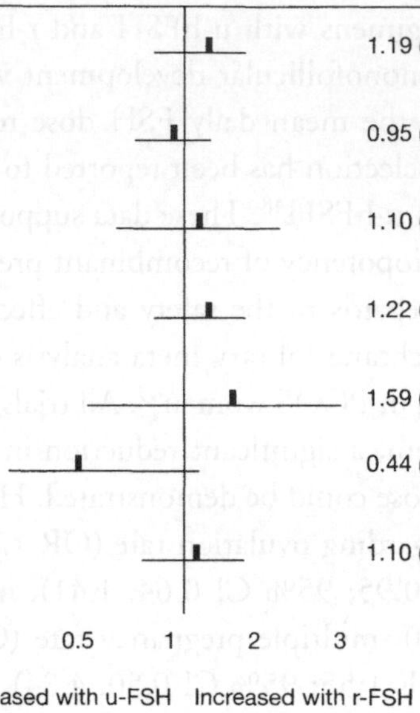

0.5   1   2   3

Increased with u-FSH   Increased with r-FSH

Figure 5.11 Summary data of outcomes for r-hFSH versus u-hFSH for ovulation induction in anovulatory women

LH therapy

Recent evidence points to a central role for LH in both steroid biosynthesis and the follicular selection and dominance process[51,52]. Two series of clinical experiments have been performed to assess the minimal and maximal doses of LH required to achieve adequate follicular growth. First, the minimal effective dose needed to complete folliculogenesis according to the 'LH threshold theory' has been tested in women with gonadotropic insufficiency (WHO group I anovulation). Second, the consequences of high doses of LH to test the 'LH ceiling concept' have been evaluated in women with WHO group II anovulation.

LH threshold

According to the two cell – two gonadotropin theory, it has been postulated that androgens produced by theca cells through LH stimulation act as precursors for estrogen production. Consequently, a minimal supply of LH (the LH threshold) is required to achieve complete folliculogenesis. Evidence to

138

support this theory was provided by studies performed in patients totally deprived of FSH and LH secretion (WHO group I). In those patients, a dose-dependent study was set up to assess the effects of different doses of r-hLH (from 0 to 225 IU) in patients treated with a low-dose FSH step-up protocol[53]. Results showed that follicular growth could be observed in all treated groups but, as regards estradiol production, a minimal daily effective dose of 75 IU was required. In addition, pregnancy was observed only in patients treated with 75 or 225 IU r-hLH. Therefore, this study fully confirmed the two cell – two gonadotropin theory whereby a threshold of LH exists to ensure complete follicular development and to achieve pregnancy.

LH ceiling

Preclinical evidence suggests that developing follicles have finite requirements for exposure to LH, beyond which normal maturation ceases[54]. Indeed, *in vitro* studies using human granulosa cells from preovulatory follicles have shown that LH exerts a dual dose-dependent effect. While LH constantly stimulates steroid production by mature granulosa cells, the effects of LH on cell proliferation are dose dependent: low LH concentrations stimulate *in vitro* cell proliferation while high doses exert a suppressive effect. These data have given rise to the concept of an 'LH ceiling', which defines an upper limit of stimulation.

This hypothesis that over-dosing with r-hLH during the late follicular phase could suppress the development of follicles was assessed in two studies performed in WHO group II anovulatory patients who over-responded to FSH[52,55]. In the first study[55], the eligibility criteria were a hyper-response to FSH treatment defined as the presence of > 4 follicles that were > 8 mm and < 13 mm in diameter. The FSH treatment was then stopped and the patients were randomized to receive placebo or two different daily doses of r-hLH (225 or 450 IU). Although the mean number of follicles of > 10 mm at the time of hCG administration tended to decrease, the difference did not achieve significance. Therefore, another prospective randomized study was conducted to evaluate the effects of larger doses of r-hLH[55]. Women with WHO group II anovulation who over-responded to FSH stimulation were selected if the number of 11–15-mm follicles was > 3, in the absence of a follicle of > 15 mm. They were then randomized to receive for a maximum of 7 days placebo or four different doses of r-hLH (7.5, 15, 30 or 60 μg; equivalent to about 165, 330, 660 and 1325 IU), while a residual daily dose of 37.5 IU of FSH was maintained. The criterion for hCG administration was no more than two follicles of ≥ 16 mm.

139

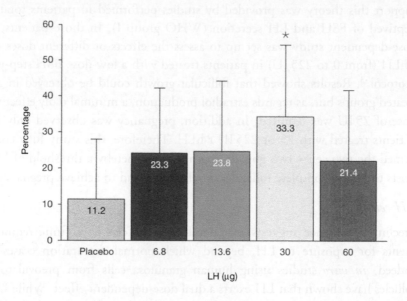

Figure 5.12 Percentage of patients who had achieved the objective of one single follicle. Those who received 30 µg r-hLH displayed a significantly higher rate of monofollicular development, adjusted to BMI and FSH dose. *$p < 0.05$

Results showed that the proportion of patients who received hCG was significantly higher in the group treated with 30 µg r-hLH (Figure 5.12). Furthermore, those patients achieved a significantly higher rate of mono-follicular ovulation. These data support the hypothesis of a ceiling effect of LH upon follicular growth. They also showed that granulosa luteinization was observed only in patients who received the highest LH dose (60 µg), confirming different LH requirements in the processes of follicular growth and granulosa cell luteinization.

hCG therapy

For the past few decades, urinary human chorionic gonadotropin (u-hCG) has been used to induce final follicular maturation and for triggering ovulation. Recombinant technology has enabled preparations that can mimic the endogenous LH surge to be developed.

A recent meta-analysis compared the cycle outcome when r-hCG and u-hCG were used[56]. No significant difference was demonstrated in induction of final follicular maturation, triggering of ovulation assessed by plasma progesterone values in the luteal phase. However, r-hCG administration was associated with a reduction in the incidence of local side-effects and other minor adverse events (OR 0.47, 95% CI 0.32, 0.70).

The ability of r-hLH to mimic the endogenous LH surge has been assessed only in women undergoing ovarian stimulation with multifollicular development for IVF or ICSI treatment. While these studies have confirmed the efficacy of r-hLH to promote oocyte maturation[57], at an effective dose of 15 000 IU r-hLH, no dose-finding studies have been performed so far to assess its ability for triggering ovulation in cycles with monofollicular development. It may be presumed that, due to the high cost of this preparation, r-hLH would not be used to trigger ovulation but would be reserved for some specific regimens with FSH co-administration during the ovarian stimulation itself, as previously discussed.

Luteal support by administration of progesterone or r-hCG is usually not required in cycles treated with gonadotropins alone. Indeed, the quality of the corpus luteum, assessed by progesterone plasma measurement, is dependent on several factors: the course of follicular development induced by FSH, the follicular rupture induced by r-hCG and the support by endogenous LH secretion in the luteal phase. Therefore, if the ovarian stimulation has been adequately driven, luteal support is not necessary, except for patients with profound LH deficiency (WHO group I anovulation). In this situation, repetitive administration of small doses of r-hCG is recommended to maintain the corpus luteum.

Adjuvant therapies

GnRH analogs

As previously mentioned, the concomitant use of GnRH agonists with gonadotropin preparations in women with PCOS did not improve the outcome of non-IVF cycles with regard to the pregnancy rate. Indeed, the incidence of moderate hyperstimulation syndrome was similar. This observation points to a primary intraovarian defect in PCOS anovulation. Some reports also indicated that co-treatment with GnRH agonist and u-hMG may reduce the miscarriage rate. Nevertheless, the role of inappropriate LH secretion in the occurrence of miscarriages has been recently challenged. Moreover, GnRH-a administration significantly increases the duration and the cost of the stimulation regimen. For these reasons, prescription of GnRH agonist should not be recommended in ovulation induction regimens, e.g.

in patients with PCOS. For those exposed to a risk of a premature LH surge, short-term use of GnRH antagonist should be preferred.

Insulin sensitizers

In another section (5.1), we have shown that insulin is of prime importance in women with PCOS. As the rate of insulin resistance is as high as 50–80% in women with PCOS, it appears that a very large proportion of cases of anovulation and infertility are associated with hyperinsulinemia.

In normogonadotropic anovulatory (WHO group II) patients, hyperinsulinemia and obesity are sometimes associated and contribute to anovulation. Loss of weight can partly restore ovulation through a reduction of insulin concentrations. In those patients with PCOS, weight reduction may also improve symptoms of hyperandrogenism (acne and hirsutism) and further restore ovulation. It should be kept in mind that a loss of just 5–10% of basal body weight may be effective in restoring reproductive function. Therefore, weight loss is the first line of treatment in any obese patient. Efforts should be made by both medical and paramedical teams to counsel these patients for lifestyle modifications.

As previously mentioned, metformin, an oral biguanide, has been shown to be effective in reducing hyperinsulinemia and, to some extent, hyperandrogenemia. It was thus assumed that metformin administration prior to FSH stimulation might be useful to reduce the risk of overstimulation. In two small studies performed in CC-resistant PCOS women, a trend towards a reduction in the number of developed follicles or in the ovulation and pregnancy rates has been reported[58,59]. In a recent study set up in insulin-resistant, normogonadotropic anovulatory women, metformin in addition to FSH therapy resulted in a higher proportion of monofollicular development[60]. These preliminary data support the hypothesis that reducing insulin levels may normalize the endocrine profile and reduce the risk of overstimulation. Further randomized controlled trials are needed to confirm these results.

Protocols for normo-ovulatory women

Ovarian stimulation associated with IUI has rapidly gained popularity over the past 15 years. Indeed, IUI has proved to be effective for some causes of infertility. Couples whose infertility is related to mild to moderate sperm abnormalities may benefit from a timely introduction of washed spermatozoa into the uterine cavity. As recently reported[61], ovarian stimulation has an independent positive effect. Indeed, the worse the semen factor the more important IUI becomes, and the better the semen factor, the more important ovarian stimulation becomes, although it is generally accepted nowadays that IUI is not the treatment of choice for moderate to severe male factor infertility but only for mild factor infertility. Therefore, ovarian stimulation is particularly relevant in patients with unexplained infertility[62]. The rationale for administering gonadotropins in women whose ovulation is usually normal is based on two findings: gonadotropin therapy is likely to overcome a subtle defect in ovarian function and to enhance the likelihood of pregnancy by increasing the number of eggs available for fertilization.

The next question to be addressed is: what should be the objective of the ovarian stimulation in terms of number of follicles? Indeed, ovarian stimulation is acceptable only when it leads to singleton pregnancy or, occasionally, twin pregnancies[63]. Recent guidelines from the National Institute of Clinical Excellence (NICE) in the UK recommend that ovarian stimulation should not be automatically offered, as it carries a high risk of multiple pregnancy.

One of the most relevant issues in clinical practice is the determination of the optimal number as well as the most adequate size of the follicles at the time of hCG administration to achieve the goal of a singleton pregnancy. In natural cycles, a follicle attains a mean diameter of 17–25 mm before ovulation. In stimulated cycles, it is more difficult to define the critical size breakpoint and there is no agreed definition of a mature-sized follicle. According to the study by Silverberg et al.[64], follicles measuring 17 mm or larger on the day of hCG administration would ovulate significantly more often (95.5% for > 20 mm, 81.2% for 19–20 mm, 72.5% for 17–18 mm) than would those follicles measuring 16 mm or lower (37.4% for 15–16 mm, 0.5% for ≤ 14 mm). However, many other clinical trials have shown that, when assessing the risk of multiple pregnancy, the number of medium-sized follicles must be considered. Presuming that each implantation derives from a follicle observed on the day of hCG administration and that the largest follicle represents the most mature, Richmond et al.[65] reported that follicles of 15 mm have an 8% chance of producing viable implantation and those of 14 mm a reduced incidence (4%) of implantaion. They suggested that tighter restriction to hCG criteria using assessments of secondary follicle diameters, based upon a critical diameter of 15 mm, may lower the multiple pregnancy rate.

Table 5.2 Cut-off values for the woman's age, estradiol values and number/size of follicles at the time of hCG administration, determined from the analysis of the ovarian stimulation leading to single or multiple pregnancies in normo-ovulatory women

	Single	Multiple	Age of patient (years)	Estradiol hCG day (pg/ml)	No. of follicles, hCG day
Navot, 1991[66]	51	51			Follicle 15–17 mm
Fahri, 1996[67]	180	28			>3 follicles ≥14 mm
Valbuena, 1996[68]	366	126	<30	>1000	>6 follicle ≥12 mm
Goldfarb, 1997[69]	78	13			Follicle >10 mm
Stone, 1999[70]	198	25			>6 follicles ≥18 mm
Pasqualotto, 1999[71]	100	22		>583	NS
Gleicher, 2000[72]	314	127		>1385	>7 follicles ≥10 mm
Dickey, 2001[73]	335	73	<35	>1000	>6 follicles ≥12 mm
Tur, 2001[74]	1477	401	≤32	>862	>3 follicles ≥10 mm
Kaplan, 2002[75]	85	14	Significant		Follicle ≥15 mm
Dickey, 2005[76]	441	146	≤37	>1000	>4 follicles ≥10 mm

Many clinical studies have been published over the past 15 years to address the issue of the optimal stimulation to achieve a pregnancy without increasing the risk of high-order multiple pregnancy (HOMP).

Different factors have been reported to be associated with a high risk of HOMP: the woman's age, serum estradiol values and the number/size of follicles. As shown in Table 5.2, there is no consensus on the limits that could be considered as acceptable in clinical practice. Indeed, published studies have demonstrated a wide range in the cut-off values for serum estradiol as well as for the number and size of follicles.

These data emphasize that multiple pregnancy might be correlated with the number of intermediate-sized follicles rather than the number of pre-ovulatory follicles. Moreover, two different clinical teams have recently published similar conclusions by analyzing predictive factors for HOMP from large series of pregnancies.

In the study by Tur et al.[74], 1878 consecutive pregnancies were retrospectively analyzed. Employing univariate, multivariate and receiver-operating characteristic analyses, a three-variable model was developed to identify patients at high risk for HOMP. It was found that the risk of HOMP was significantly increased in women with more than three follicles of ≥10 mm, serum estradiol values of >862 pg/ml and age ≤32 years. Moreover, the effectiveness in clinical practice of such a prediction model has been determined in a series of 849 consecutive infertile patients undergoing a total of 1542 treatment cycles[77]. The authors reported that the use of a prediction model implying cancellation of all cycles at high risk of HOMP would result in an 8% (95% CI 6.8, 9.2%) reduction in pregnancy rate but also in 285% (95% CI 279, 291%) reduction of HOMP. Therefore, it is possible to maintain a low risk of HOMP with a good pregnancy rate in normo-ovulatory patients receiving gonadotropin in an IUI program.

Interestingly, these data are in accordance with another recent study from the USA where stimulation regimens are usually more aggressive than in Europe and where HOMP is not currently considered as a side-effect of ovarian stimulation. Indeed, Dickey et al.[76] also reported that HOMP could be predicted by age (32 years), serum estradiol values (1000 pg/ml), number of follicles of diameter ≥10 mm (4) and number of treated cycles (<3). The authors concluded that the use of controlled ovarian stimulation (COH) rather than minimal stimulation to increase the probability of pregnancy is unnecessary and increases the incidence of HOMP without increasing overall possibility of the patient becoming pregnant.

Interestingly, other authors recently challenged the principle of stimulation on the observation that mild stimulation does not result in higher pregnancy rates than IUI in the natural cycle while increasing the rate of HOMP[78]. They stated that there is no place for the use of gonadotropin in IUI treatment. However, in this study, criteria for cycle cancellation were relatively liberal (six follicles ≥14 mm). Therefore, these data emphasize that less aggressive regimens of FSH administration and stricter criteria to trigger ovulation are required when it comes to ovarian stimulation in normo-ovulatory women. Furthermore, they pointed out the need for better standardization in ultrasound reports and for reducing intra- and interobserver

Table 5.3 Protocols used for ovarian stimulation in normo-ovulatory women				
	Protocol	Criteria for cancellation	Pregnancy rate (%)	Multiple pregnancy rate (%)
Balasch, 1994[79]	75 IU FSH/day from D7	None	13	0
Gregoriou, 1995[80]	75 IU hMG/day from D3 step-up	>4 follicles ≥16 mm E2 >450 pg/ml	25.7	9.1 (twins only)
Cohlen, 1998[81]	75 IU FSH/day from D3 step-up	>3 follicles ≥18 mm E2 >1800 pg/ml	13.7	9.5 (twins only)
Guzick, 1999[82]	150 IU FSH/day fixed dose from D3	E2 >3000 pg/ml	9	25 (including HOMP)
Goverde, 2000[83]	75 IU FSH/day from D3 step-up	>3 follicles ≥18 mm >6 follicles ≥14 mm	8.7	29 (twins only)
Papageorgiou, 2004[84]	50–75 IU FSH from D4	>2 follicles ≥15 mm	10	8 (twins mainly)
Ragni, 2004[85]	50 IU FSH from D3 GnRH antagonist	>2 follicles ≥15 mm	36.6	0
E2, estradiol; D, day; HOMP, high-order multiple pregnancy				

variability to reduce the confounding factors of ultrasonographic follicular assessment.

Thus, the choice of ovarian stimulation regimen is crucial to achieve the objective of a singleton pregnancy. Nevertheless, few studies have been performed so far to determine the best protocol (Table 5.3). Interestingly, protocols with low FSH doses similar to those recommended in anovulatory patients have been used in women with ovulatory cycles. More recently, it has been shown that minimal ovarian stimulation with r-hFSH (50–75 IU/day) from day 4 to 7 with subsequent adjustment of FSH doses may reduce the rates of twins while maintaining acceptable pregnancy rates[84]. Addition of a GnRH antagonist when the leading follicle reaches a diameter of 14 mm has been proposed[85] in women treated with two different regimens of low doses of r-hFSH (50 IU daily or on alternate days) before IUI. The potential benefit of a GnRH antagonist in an IUI program is better control of the timing of insemination. In this small series of patients, a daily dose of r-hFSH proved to be more efficient to achieve a pregnancy but the value of the GnRH antagonist *per se* has not been assessed.

Therefore, prospective studies are required to determine the optimal regimen to achieve a limited number of follicular developments in women with ovulatory cycles. It must be kept in mind that a brief but distinct elevation of FSH levels above the threshold in the early follicular phase actually increases the number of small antral follicles[86]. In contrast, a moderate but continued elevation of FSH levels during the mid- to late follicular phase interferes with a single dominant follicle and induces ongoing growth of multiples follicles. Therefore, it is likely that manipulation of exogenous FSH should be restricted to a limited period of the follicular phase with a conservative use of gonadotropins.

CONCLUSION

Gonadotropin therapy has proved to be highly effective to achieve singleton live birth in women suffering from chronic anovulation. Indeed, during the past two decades, many advances in ovarian physiology and in the manufacture of gonadotropins have improved the efficacy, efficiency and safety of ovarian stimulation regimens. The following guidelines may help physicians achieve the objective of a singleton live birth.

(1) Initial patient characteristics are able to predict the chances of treatment response and outcome. Prediction models are available to define the FSH starting dose.

(2) The objective of the ovarian stimulation in terms of number of follicles must be defined according to the infertility context.

(3) A stepwise (step-up and step-down) administration of FSH is required to reduce the risk of multifollicular development.

(4) A strict application of criteria to trigger ovulation or to cancel the cycle is needed.

(5) Improvements in product purity, consistency and delivery have been achieved for recombinant FSH and LH preparations. Furthermore, they can be used separately to mimic the physiological events of the menstrual cycle.

(6) The use of GnRH analogs is not helpful in preventing the risk of multifollicular development.

(7) Addition of insulin sensitizers should be considered in patients with some degree of insulin resistance.

Further refinements in ovarian stimulation regimens are needed to improve both efficacy and safety. Individualization of ovulation stimulation protocols is likely to be the most important factor in preventing the risk of HOMP.

When gonadotropins are also used in normo-ovulatory women undergoing IUI, the risk of multiple pregnancy is much higher. Protocols to obtain a limited number of growing follicles should be better defined.

Because 'classical' induction of ovulation strategies in anovulatory patients has been experienced by some authors as a time-consuming treatment modality, patients are increasingly offered 'controlled ovarian stimulation' combined with IUI or IVF as the first-line therapy. However, this strategy is not based on sound scientific evidence and will increase overall treatment cost[87].

5.3 Aromatase inhibitors

INTRODUCTION

As previously discussed in another section of this book, the first-line therapy in patients with chronic anovulation during the past 40 years has been CC. While being effective in inducing ovulation in selected patients, comfortable and convenient because of its oral administration, relatively safe and inexpensive, this medication may have adverse effects mainly related to its anti-estrogenic effects on cervical mucus and the endometrium. These effects could explain, at least in part, the differences seen between ovulation rates and pregnancy rates in CC-responsive patients.

These drawbacks of CC treatment opened the field for another medication: orally active and without antiestrogenic side-effects. The recent availability of a new generation of specific aromatase inhibitors (AIs), initially used for patients with breast cancer for their suppressive effects on estradiol synthesis, led to the initiation of studies assessing the potential effect of AIs in inducing ovulation.

AIs can be steroidal or non-steroidal compounds that suppress estrogen biosynthesis by blocking the action of the enzyme aromatase, which converts androstenedione to estrone, and testosterone to estradiol.

The third generation of commercially available AIs has been developed to reduce the side-effects reported with first and second generation AIs, and to improve potency and specificity in inhibiting the aromatase enzyme.

Anastrazole and letrozole are non-steroidal, reversible, competitive AIs with high potency to reduce estrogen levels. These AIs are completely absorbed after oral administration, with a mean terminal half-life of about 45 hours (range 30–60 hours).

MECHANISM OF ACTION

As regards ovulation induction, it was speculated that the loss of estrogen synthesis induced by AIs in patients with preserved estrogen synthesis should be able to overcome the negative feedback effect of estrogen at the hypothalamic–pituitary level. The resultant increase in gonadotropin secretion should stimulate follicular growth and induce ovulation.

As compared with CC, which binds to estrogen receptors (ERs) throughout the body for an extended period of time and results in major depletion without replenishment of ERs, AIs do not deplete ERs. Therefore, several advantages of AIs have been postulated:

(1) A shorter half-life (about 45 hours) to reduce a long-term effect and the incidence of side-effects.

(2) Preserved ER function at the pituitary level: thus, the feedback effect of stimulated estradiol levels on FSH pituitary secretion remains intact and results in suppression of endogenous FSH secretion in the late follicular phase. As a consequence, the FSH window can be closed, leading to atresia of secondary follicles and to a higher rate of monofollicular ovulation (Figure 5.13).

(3) The absence of peripheral side-effects, mainly on cervical mucus and endometrium. It has even been speculated that the suppression of endogenous estrogen synthesis induced by AIs may result in upregulation of ERs at the endometrium level with higher sensitivity to estradiol. This should lead to rapid endometrial growth once estrogen secretion is restored and to better endometrial development and thickness.

(4) The intraovarian increase in androgen concentration which stimulates FSH receptor synthesis within granulosa cells of primates could participate in the increased follicular sensitivity to FSH and improve the effectiveness of AIs to stimulate follicular growth, with small doses.

INDICATION

In relation to their mechanism of action, AIs – in the same way as CC – must be strictly prescribed to anovulatory women whose endogenous estrogen secretion is preserved. In clinical practice, these women can be easily

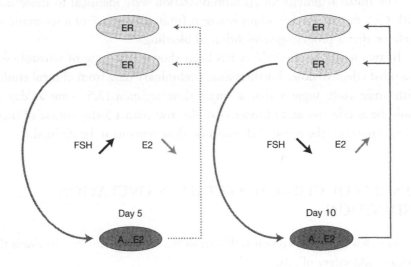

Figure 5.13 At the early stage of the follicular phase, aromatase inhibitor administration induces a rise in serum follicle stimulating hormone (FSH) concentrations related to a decrease in serum estradiol (E2) concentrations. Thereafter, simultaneously with follicular growth, serum E2 levels increase. Owing to the preserved physiological feedback of E2 at the hypothalamic–pituitary level, serum FSH concentration decreases and monofollicular development can be expected. A, androgen; ER, estrogen receptor

identified by the occurrence of bleeding following short-term progestogen administration (progestogen challenge test). Therefore, women with WHO group II anovulation, including polycystic ovary syndrome (PCOS) patients, are particularly prone to be responsive to AIs.

As previously reported with CC, AIs may also be used as an adjunct to exogenous FSH or other medications to improve the outcome of controlled ovarian stimulation.

PROTOCOLS

In most studies looking at the clinical applications of AIs in ovulation-induction protocols, the daily doses used were identical to those commonly prescribed in breast cancer, which have been demonstrated to provide optimal reduction of E2 production. In the case of letrozole (Femara®, Novartis Pharmaceuticals), the dose used is 2.5 mg/day. In the case of anastrazole (Arimidex®, AstraZeneca Pharmaceuticals), the dose is 1 mg/day.

The initial regimens for AI administration were identical to those used with CC, that is a 5-day administration from days 3 to 7 of a spontaneous cycle or after a progestogen-withdrawal bleeding.

In two recent studies[88,89], it has been shown that 5 mg of letrozole was the most effective dose. Furthermore, preliminary data from clinical studies with anastrazole suggest that a single dose regimen (2.5–5 mg at day 3) could be as effective as and more cost-effective than a 5-day course of treatment. However, the optimal therapeutic dose remains to be defined.

RESULTS OF CLINICAL STUDIES IN OVULATION INDUCTION

To date, few randomized controlled trials have been performed to assess the efficacy and safety of AIs.

The first trial with AIs for inducing ovulation was conducted in women who did not ovulate with CC[90]. AIs were first prescribed for 5 consecutive days, typically from day 3 to day 7 of the menstrual cycle. Further studies were conducted in a limited number of anovulatory women who failed to respond to CC or women with unexplained infertility[91]. The overall conclusion was that a 5-day course of treatment with letrozole (2.5 mg/day, from cycle day 3 to day 7) was as effective as CC (50–100 mg/day for 5 days) for inducing ovulation. Interestingly, peak E2 levels on the day of human chorionic gonadotropin (hCG) administration were reduced by almost 50% in the AI group in spite of the presence of an almost similar number of growing and maturing follicles (about two follicles).

Other studies were performed to test the effects of combined AI–FSH/hMG regimens. The aim of sequential or overlapping administration of AIs and gonadotropins was to obtain controlled ovarian hyperstimulation in patients with unexplained infertility (Figure 5.14). The results showed an almost identical number of follicles (about three) recruited, and mature follicles. A trend toward a further reduction in FSH needs was encountered in the AI–FSH group, as compared with the CC–FSH group[92]. The observation of a thicker endometrium in the AI–FSH group (9.1 ± 0.2 mm) as compared with the CC–FSH group (8.0 ± 0.2 mm) supports the contention that different endometrial effects of AI and CC were instrumental in achieving higher pregnancy rates in the AI–FSH group. It was also reported that E2 levels were markedly lower in the AI–FSH group (about half as high) as compared with both FSH only and CC–FSH groups,

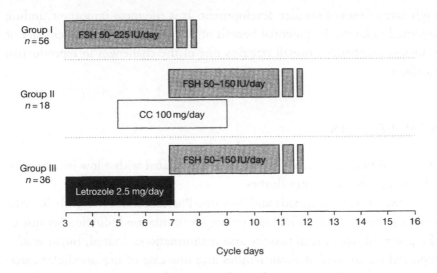

Figure 5.14 Use of follicle stimulating hormone (FSH), aromatase inhibitors (AIs) and clomiphene citrate (CC) in unexplained infertility. Experimental diagram of a prospective trial including three study groups, using FSH alone (group I), CC and FSH (group II) and AI and FSH (group III). Adapted from reference 90

while ovulation occurred spontaneously in > 50% of women receiving CC–FSH or AI–FSH. In these patients, pregnancy rates were comparable with those observed in women in whom ovulation was artificially triggered with exogenous hCG.

The reduction in the FSH dose required led to studies assessing the benefits of AIs in patients with a poor response to FSH. Preliminary results tend to show a slight improvement in the ovarian response[93]. Further studies are required to assess its effectiveness when compared with the CC–FSH regimen.

As regards the pregnancy outcome, a recent report[91] described a cohort study comparing the outcome of pregnancies achieved after letrozole (2.5 or 5 mg alone or with gonadotropins – 133 pregnancies) and other ovarian stimulation regimens (CC ± gonadotropins – 133 pregnancies or gonadotropins alone – 110 pregnancies) with a control group of spontaneous pregnancies. AI treatment was associated with comparable miscarriage and ectopic pregnancy rates compared with other groups including spontaneous conception. More importantly, letrozole use was associated with a significant reduction in multiple gestation rate compared with CC (4.3 vs. 22%, respectively). This latter result is consistent with the concept of an intact negative feedback loop with AI treatments and with previous reports of the high rate of monofollicular development. It is the most important finding reported so far on the potential benefit of AIs, because the high incidence of multiple pregnancies overall remains one of the challenges in reproductive medicine.

SIDE-EFFECTS

In clinical practice, AIs are generally well tolerated with a low incidence of adverse effects such as hot flushes.

However, Health Canada and Novartis Pharmaceuticals recently issued a warning that letrozole should not be used for ovulation induction because of the potential risk of fetal toxicity and malformations. Indeed, Biljan *et al.*[94] reported six congenital abnormalities and one case of hepatocellular carcinoma among 150 births resulting from the use of letrozole for ovulation induction at the ASRM meeting in 2005. Moreover, they observed a significant increase in locomotor and cardiac abnormalities in the letrozole-treated pregnancies compared with controls. Although these findings need to be confirmed in a large-scale study, they emphasize that letrozole should not be used routinely but only within randomized clinical trials. It should be noted that these findings cannot be translated to other AIs but refer specifically to letrozole. For anastrazole, no teratogenic effects have been reported.

CONCLUSION

Although to date CC is still the first-line treatment of anovulatory disorders, it is likely that in the near future AIs could replace CC. Compared with CC AIs offer several advantages due to the fact that they do not directly interfere with the ER. Therefore, the physiological negative feedback effect of estrogen on pituitary FSH secretion is intact, with the potential advantage of a high rate of monofollicular ovulation and a reduced risk of multiple pregnancies. Moreover, the absence of peripheral antiestrogenic side-effects may lead to a higher pregnancy rate compared with that found in CC-treated women.

However, further randomized controlled trials are required to confirm the preliminary data reported by the limited number of clinical trials to date.

More importantly, a worldwide survey is required to assess the global risk of teratogenic effects of AIs.

REFERENCES

1. Greenblatt RB, Bafrield WE, Jungck EC, et al. Induction of ovulation with MRL/41. Preliminary report. JAMA 1961; 178: 101–4
2. Adashi EY. Clomiphene citrate: mechanism(s) and site(s) of action – a hypothesis revisited. Fertil Steril 1984; 42: 331–44
3. Rostami-Hodjegan A, Lennard MS, Tucker GT, et al. Monitoring plasma concentrations to individualize treatment with clomiphene citrate. Fertil Steril 2004; 81: 1187–93
4. Homburg R. Clomiphene citrate – end of an era? A mini-review. Hum Reprod 2005; 8: 2043–51
5. Macgregor AH, Johnson JE, Bunde CA. Further clinical experience with clomiphene citrate. Fertil Steril 1968; 19: 616–22
6. Garcia J, Jones GS, Wentz AC. The use of clomiphene citrate. Fertil Steril 1977; 28: 707–17
7. Gysler M, March CM, Mishell DR, et al. A decade's experience with an individualized clomiphene treatment regimen including its effect on the postcoital test. Fertil Steril 1982; 37: 161–7
8. Hammond MG. Monitoring techniques for improved pregnancy rates during clomiphene ovulation induction. Fertil Steril 1984; 42: 499–509
9. Kousta E, White DM, Frank S. Modern use of clomiphene citrate in induction of ovulation. Hum Reprod Update 1997; 3: 359–65
10. Messinis IE, Milingos SD. Future use of clomiphene in ovarian stimulation. Clomiphene in the 21st century. Hum Reprod 1998; 13: 2362–5
11. Imani B, Eijkemans MJ, te Velde ER, et al. A nomogram to predict the probability of live birth after clomiphene citrate induction of ovulation in normogonadotropic oligo-amenorrheic infertility. Fertil Steril 2002; 77: 91–7
12. Van Santbrink EJP, Eijkemans MJ, Laven JSE, et al. Patient-tailored conventional ovulation induction algorithms in anovulatory infertility. Trends Endocrinol Metab 2005; 16: 381–9
13. Imani B, Eijkemans MJ, te Velde ER, et al. Predictors of patients remaining anovulatory during clomiphene citrate induction of ovulation in normogonadotropic oligo-amenorrheic infertility. J Clin Endocrinol Metab 1998; 83: 2361–5
14. Kurabayashi T, Suzuki M, Fujita K, et al. Prognostic factors for ovulatory response with clomiphene citrate in polycystic ovary syndrome. Eur J Obstet Gynecol Reprod Biol 2006; 126: 201–5
15. Attia GR, Rainey WE, Carr BR. Metformin directly inhibits androgen production in human thecal cells. Fertil Steril 2001; 76: 517–24
16. Mansfield R, Galea R, Brincat M et al. Metformin has direct effects on human ovarian steroidogenesis. Fertil Steril 2003; 79: 956–62
17. Lord JM, Flight IH, Norman RJ. Insulin-sensitising drugs (metformin, troglitazone, rosiglitazone, pioglitazone, D-chiro-inositol) for polycystic ovary syndrome. Cochrane Database Syst Rev 2003; (3): CD003053

18. Kashyap S, Wells GA, Rosenwaks Z. Insulin-sensitizing agents as primary therapy for patients with polycystic ovarian syndrome. Hum Reprod 2004; 19: 2474–83
19. The Practice Committee of the American Society for Reproductive Medicine. Use of clomiphene citrate in women. Fertil Steril 2003; 80: 1302–8
20. Steiner AZ, Terplan M, Paulson RJ. Comparison of tamoxifen and clomiphene citrate for ovulation induction: a meta-analysis. Hum Reprod 2005; 20: 1511–15
21. Ness RB, Cramer DW, Goodman MT, et al. Infertility, fertility drug, and ovarian cancer: a pooled analysis of case–control studies. Am J Epidemiol 2002; 155: 217–24
22. Guzick DS, Sullivan MW, Adamson GD, et al. Efficacy of treatment for unexplained infertility. Fertil Steril 1998; 70: 207–13
23. Hughes E, Collins I, Van de Kerckhove P. Clomiphene citrate for unexplained subfertility in women. Cochrane Database Syst Rev 2000; (3): CD000057
24. Chappel SC. Heterogeneity of FSH: control and physiological function. Hum Reprod Update 1995; 1: 479–87
25. Hugues JN. Recombinant human FSH: a scientific step to clinical improvement. Reprod BioMed Online 2001; 2: 54–64
26. Brown JB. Pituitary control of ovarian function – concepts derived from gonadotropin therapy. Aust NZ J Obstet Gynaecol 1978; 18: 46–54
27. Baird DT. A model for follicular selection and ovulation: lessons from superovulation. J Ster Biochem 1987; 27: 15–23
28. Macklon NS, Fauser BCJM. Follicle-stimulating hormone and advanced follicle development in the human. Arch Med Res 2001; 32: 595–600
29. Fauser BC, Van Heusden AM. Manipulation of human ovarian function: physiological concepts and clinical consequences. Endocr Rev 1997; 18: 71–106
30. Homburg R, Levy T, Ben-Rafael Z. A comparative prospective study of conventional regimen with chronic low-dose administration of follicle-stimulating hormone for anovulation associated with polycystic ovary syndrome. Fertil Steril 1995; 63: 729–33
31. Hedon B, Hugues JN, Emperaire JC, et al. A comparative prospective study of a chronic low dose versus a conventional ovulation stimulation regimen using recombinant human follicle stimulating hormone in anovulatory infertile women. Hum Reprod 1998; 13: 2688–92
32. Homburg R, Insler V. Ovulation induction in perspective. Hum Reprod Update 2002; 8: 449–62
33. Homburg R, Howles CM. Low-dose FSH therapy for anovulatory infertility associated with polycystic ovary syndrome: rationale, results, reflections and refinements. Hum Reprod Update 1999; 5: 493–9
34. Van der Meer M, Hompes PG, Scheele F, et al. The importance of endogenous feedback for monofollicular growth in low-dose step-up ovulation induction with follicle-stimulating hormone in polycystic ovary syndrome: a randomized study. Fertil Steril 1996; 66: 571–6
35. Nugent D, Vandekerckhove P, Hughes E, et al. Gonadotropin therapy for ovulation induction in subfertility associated with polycystic ovary syndrome. Cochrane Database Systematic Rev 2000; (4): CD000410
36. White DM, Polson DW, Kiddy D, et al. Induction of ovulation with low-dose gonadotropins in polycystic ovary syndrome: an analysis of 109 pregnancies in 225 women. J Clin Endocrinol Metab 1996; 81: 3821–4
37. Hugues JN, Cedrin-Durnerin I, Avril C, et al. Sequential step-up and step-down dose regimen: an alternative method for ovulation induction with follicle-stimulating hormone in polycystic ovarian syndrome. Hum Reprod 1996; 11: 2581–4

38. Balasch J, Fabregues F, Creus M, et al. Recombinant human follicle-stimulating hormone for ovulation induction in polycystic ovary syndrome: a prospective, randomized trial of two starting doses in a chronic low-dose step-up protocol. J Assist Reprod Genet 2000; 17: 561–5

39. Ares-Serono. A phase III, open, randomized, multicentre study to compare the safety and efficacy of recombinant human follicle stimulating hormone (Gonal-F) administered subcutaneously with that of urinary human follicle stimulating hormone (Metrodin) given intramuscularly, to induce ovulation in WHO Group II anovulatory infertile women. Ares-Serono, Internal Report, 1995

40. Van Santbrink EJ, Donderwinkel PF, van Dessel TJ, et al. Gonadotropin induction of ovulation using a step-down dose regimen: single-centre clinical experience in 82 patients. Hum Reprod 1995; 10: 1048–53

41. Van Santbrink EJ, Fauser BCJM. Urinary follicle-stimulating hormone for normogonadotropic clomiphene-resistant anovulatory infertility: prospective, randomized comparison between low dose step-up and step-down dose regimens. J Clin Endocrinol Metab 1997; 82: 3597–602

42. Balasch J, Fabregues F, Creus M, et al. Follicular development and hormone concentrations following recombinant FSH administration for anovulation associated with polycystic ovarian syndrome: prospective, randomized comparison between low-dose step-up and modified step-down regimens. Hum Reprod 2001; 16: 652–6

43. Christin-Maitre S, Hugues JN, on behalf of the Recombinant FSH Study Group. A comparative randomized multicentric study comparing the step-up versus step-down protocol in polycystic ovary syndrome. Hum Reprod 2003; 18: 1626–31

44. Imani B, Eijkemans MJ, Faessen GH, et al. Prediction of the individual follicle-stimulating hormone threshold for gonadotropin induction of ovulation in normogonadotropic anovulatory infertility: an approach to increase safety and efficiency. Fertil Steril 2002; 77: 83–90

45. Mulders AG, Eijkemans MJ, Imani B, et al. A prediction of chances for success or complications in gonadotropin ovulation induction in normogonadotrophic anovulatory infertility. Reprod BioMed Online 2003; 7: 170–8

46. Mulders AG, Laven JS, Eijkemans MJ, et al. Patient predictors for outcome of gonadotropin ovulation induction in women with normogonadotrophic anovulatory infertility: a meta-analysis. Hum Reprod Update 2003; 9: 429–49

47. Hughes EG, Collins JA. Ovulation induction with urinary FSH versus HMG for clomiphene-resistant polycystic ovary syndrome. Cochrane Review In Cochrane Library, 1996; (3)

48. Hugues JN, Bstandig B, Bry-Gauillard H, et al. Comparison of the effectiveness of recombinant and urinary FSH preparations in the achievement of follicular selection in chronic anovulation. Reprod BioMed Online 2001; 3: 195–8

49. Van Wely M, Bayram N, van der Veen M. Recombinant FSH in alternative doses or versus urinary gonadotropins for ovulation induction in subfertility associated with polycystic ovary syndrome: a systematic review based on a Cochrane review. Hum Reprod 2003; 18: 1143–9

50. Yeko T, Pasqualini SR, Alam V, et al. Cumulative ovulation and pregnancy rates according to recombinant human FSH dosing: comparison of a new formulation of follitropin alpha in vials versus the standard formulation of follitropin alpha in ampoules. Fertil Steril 2004; 82 (Suppl 2): S119

51. Shoham Z. The clinical therapeutic window for luteinizing hormone in controlled ovarian stimulation. Fertil Steril 2002; 7: 1170–7

52. Loumaye E, Engrand P, Shoham Z, et al. Clinical evidence for an LH 'ceiling' effect induced by administration of recombinant human LH during the late follicular phase of stimulated cycles in World Health Organization type I and type II anovulation. Hum Reprod 2003; 18: 314–22

53. The European Recombinant LH Study Group. Recombinant human LH to support recombinant FSH induced follicular development in LH and FSH deficient anovulatory women: a dose finding study. J Clin Endocrinol Metab 1998; 83: 1507–14

54. Hillier SG. Current concepts of the roles of follicle stimulating hormone and luteinizing hormone in folliculogenesis. Hum Reprod 1994; 9: 188–91

55. Hugues JN, Soussis J, Calderon I, et al. Does the addition of recombinant luteinising hormone (r-hLH) in WHO Group II anovulatory women over-responding to FSH treatment reduce the number of developing follicles? A dose finding study. Hum Reprod 2005; 20: 629–35

56. Al-Inany HG, Aboulghar M, Mansour R, et al. Recombinant versus urinary human chorionic gonadotropin for ovulation induction in assisted conception. Cochrane Database Syst Rev 2005; (2): CD003719

57. The European Recombinant LH Study Group. Recombinant human LH is as effective as, but safer than urinary human chorionic gonadotropin in inducing final follicular maturation and ovulation in IVF procedures: results of a multicenter double blind study. J Clin Endocrinol Metab 2001; 86: 2607–18

58. De Leo V, La Marca A, Ditto A, et al. Effects of metformin on gonadotropin-induced ovulation in women with polycystic ovary syndrome. Fertil Steril 1999; 72: 282–5

59. Yarali H, Yildiz BO, Demirol A, et al. Co-administration of metformin during rFSH treatment in patients with clomiphene citrate-resistant polycystic ovarian syndrome: a prospective randomized trial. Hum Reprod 2002; 17: 289–94

60. Van Santbrink EJ, Hohmann FP, Eijkemans MJC, et al. Does metformin modify ovarian responsiveness during exogenous FSH ovulation induction in normogonadotrophic anovulation? A placebo-controlled double-blind assessment. Eur J Endocrinol 2005; 152: 611–17

61. Cohlen BJ. Should we continue performing intrauterine insemination in the year 2004? Gynaecol Obstet Invest 2004; 59: 3–13

62. Hughes EG. The effectiveness of ovulation induction and intrauterine insemination in the treatment of persistent infertility: a meta-analysis. Hum Reprod 1997; 12: 1865–72

63. Balasch J. Gonadotropin ovarian stimulation and intrauterine insemination for unexplained infertility. Reprod Biomed Online 2004; 6: 664–72

64. Silverberg KM, Olive DL, Burns WN, et al. Follicular size at the time of human chorionic gonadotropin administration predicts ovulation outcome in human menopausal gonadotropin-stimulated cycles. Fertil Steril 1991; 56: 296–300

65. Richmond JR, Deshpande N, Lyall H, et al. Follicular diameters in conception cycles with and without multiple pregnancy after stimulated ovulation induction. Hum Reprod 2005; 20: 756–60

66. Navot D, Golstein N, Mor-Josef S, et al. Multiple pregnancies: risk factors and prognostic variables during induction of ovulation with human menopausal gonadotropins. Hum Reprod 1991: 6: 1152–5

67. Fahri J, West C, Patel A, et al. Treatment of anovulatory infertility. The problem of multiple pregnancy. Hum Reprod 1996; 11: 429–34

68. Valbuena D, Simon C, Romero JL, et al. Factors responsible for multiple pregnancies after ovarian stimulation and intrauterine insemination with gonadotropins. J Assist Reprod Genet 1996; 13: 663–8

69. Goldfarb JM, Peskin B, Austin C, et al. Evaluation of predictive factors for multiple pregnancies during gonadotropin/IUI treatment. J Assist Reprod Genet 1997: 14: 88–91

70. Stone BA, Vargyas M, Ringler GE et al. Determinants of the outcome of intrauterine insemination: analysis of outcomes of 9963 consecutive cycles. Am J Obstet Gynecol 1999; 180: 1522–34

71. Pasqualotto EB, Falcone T, Goldberg JM, et al. Risk factors for multiple gestation in women undergoing intrauterine insemination with ovarian stimulation. Fertil Steril 1999; 72: 613–18

72. Gleicher N, Oleske DM, Kur-Kaspa I, et al. Reducing the risk of high-order multiple pregnancy after ovarian stimulation with gonadotropins. N Engl J Med 2000; 343: 2–7

73. Dickey RP, Taylor SN, Lu PY, et al. Relationship of follicle numbers and oestradiol levels of multiple implantation in 3,608 intrauterine insemination cycles. Fertil Steril 2001; 75: 69–78

74. Tur R, Barri PN, Coroleu B, et al. Risk factors for high-order multiple implantation after ovarian stimulation with gonadotropins: evidence from a large series of 1879 consecutive pregnancies in a single centre. Hum Reprod 2001; 16: 2124–9

75. Kaplan PF, Patel M, Austin DJ, et al. Assessing the risk of multiple gestation in gonadotropin intrauterine insemination cycles. Am J Obstet Gynecol 2002; 186: 1244–9

76. Dickey RP, Taylor SN, Lu PY, et al. Risk factors for high-order multiple pregnancy and multiple birth after controlled ovarian hyperstimulation: results of 4062 intra-uterine insemination cycles. Fertil Steril 2005; 83: 671–83

77. Tur R, Barri PN, Coroleu B, et al. Use of a prediction model for high-order multiple implantation after ovarian stimulation with gonadotropins. Fertil Steril 2005; 83: 116–21

78. Goverde AJ, Lambalck CB, McDonnell J, et al. Further consideration on natural or mild stimulation cycles for intra-uterine insemination treatment: effects on pregnancy and multiple pregnancy rates. Hum Reprod 2005; 20: 3141–6

79. Balasch J, Ballesca JL, Pimentel C, et al. Late low dose pure FSH for ovarian stimulation in intra-uterine insemination cycles. Hum Reprod 1994; 9: 1863–6

80. Gregoriou G, Vitoratos N, Papadias C, et al. Controlled ovarian hyperstimlation with or without intrauterine insemination for the treatment of unexplained infertility. Int J Gynaecol Obstet 1995; 48: 55–9

81. Cohlen BJ, te Velde ER, van Kooij RJ, et al. Controlled ovarian hyperstimulation and intrauterine insemination for treating male subfertility: a controlled study. Hum Reprod 1998; 13: 1553–8

82. Guzick DS, Carson SA, Overstreet JW, et al. Efficacy of superovulation and intrauterine insemination in the treatment of infertility. N Engl J Med 1999; 340: 177–83

83. Goverde AJ, McDonnell J, Vermeiden JPW, et al. Intrauterine insemination or in vitro fertilisation in idiopathic subfertility and male subfertility: a randomised trial and cost-effectiveness analysis. Lancet 2000; 355: 13–18

84. Papageorgiou TC, Guibert J, Savale M, et al. Low dose recombinant FSH treatment may reduce multiple gestations caused by controlled ovarian stimulation and intrauterine insemination. Br J Obstet Gynaecol 2004; 111: 1277–82

85. Ragni G, Alagna F, Brigante C, et al. GnRH antagonists and mild ovarian stimulation for intrauterine insemination: a randomized study comparing different gonadotropin dosages. Hum Reprod 2004; 19: 54–8

86. Schipper I, Hop WCJ, Fauser BCJM. The FSH threshold/window concept examined by different interventions with exogenous FSH during the follicular phase of the

normal menstrual cycle: duration rather than magnitude of FSH increase affects follicle development. J Clin Endocrinol Metab 1998; 83: 1292–8

87. Van Santbrink EJ, Fauser BCJM. Is there a future for ovulation induction in the current era of assisted reproduction? Hum Reprod 2003; 18: 2499–502

88. Biljan MM, Tan SL, Tulandi T. Prospective randomized trial comparing the effects of 2.5 and 5.0 mg of letrozole (LE) on follicular development, endometrial thickness and pregnancy rate in patients undergoing super-ovulation. Fertil Steril 2002; 78: S55

89. Healey S, Tan SL, Tulandi T, et al. Effects of letrozole on superovulation with gonadotropins in women undergoing intrauterine insemination. Fertil Steril 2003; 80: 1325–9

90. Mitwally MFM, Casper RF. Use of an aromatase inhibitor for induction of ovulation in patients with an inadequate response to clomiphene citrate. Fertil Steril 2001; 75: 305–9

91. Mitwally MFM, Biljan MM, Casper RF. Pregnancy outcome after the use of an aromatase inhibitor for ovarian stimulation Am J Obstet Gynecol 2005; 192: 381–6

92. Mitwally MFM, Casper RF. Aromatase inhibition reduces gonadotropin dose required for controlled ovarian stimulation in women with unexplained infertility. Hum Reprod 2003; 18: 1588–97

93. Mitwally MFM, Casper RF. Aromatase inhibition improves ovarian response to follicle-stimulating hormone in poor responders. Fertil Steril 2002; 77: 776–80

94. Biljan MM, Hemmings R, Brassard N. The outcome of 150 babies following the treatment with letrozole or letrozole and gonadotropins. Fertil Steril 2005; 84 (Suppl 1): S95

6

Intrauterine insemination

INTRODUCTION

Intrauterine insemination (IUI) is a widely used procedure. There is some debate about whether this method should be seen as a conservative or an invasive approach. Owing to the fact that IUI does not imply extracorporeal fertilization and that usually less 'aggressive' ovarian stimulation is applied, most people nowadays see IUI as a conservative treatment option.

In the era of rapid development of assisted reproductive technologies (ART), such as *in vitro* fertilization (IVF) and intracytoplasmic sperm injection (ICSI), the question arises as to whether there is still a place for IUI as a treatment of infertility. Some experts take the position that in principle all couples should be offered either IVF or ICSI primarily, as chances for achieving a pregnancy are considerably higher for both of these methods compared with IUI. Furthermore, today in most regions around the world couples are willing to take risks and bear financial burdens in order to become pregnant within a relatively short period of time. However, the following points should be considered:

- According to good clinical practice (GCP) the physician should discuss with the couple all therapeutic options including side-effects, risks and potential costs

- Owing to the more 'invasive' character of IVF/ICSI compared with IUI it must be considered whether the couple should be exposed to these risks if other options are available

• If possible, information should be given on the basis of results from high-quality trials, when they are available

RATIONALE FOR IUI AND INDICATIONS FOR TREATMENT

The rationale for performing IUI is to increase the chances for a pregnancy by bringing a high number of good-quality sperm (normal motility, normal morphology) to the site of fertilization.

Currently proposed indications for IUI include unexplained infertility, cervical factor, mild impairment of semen quality and others. In order to demonstrate the efficacy of IUI, it would need to be compared with (timed) intercourse, and randomized trials to show a benefit of IUI for each of the indications listed would need to be performed. However, despite the widespread clinical use of this technique prospective randomized data to determine its therapeutic value are sparse compared with data on IVF/ICSI. A number of variables determine success rates of IUI, e.g. the use or non-use of ovarian stimulation, the number of inseminations per treatment cycle, different methods of timing ovulation, different sites of insemination and various methods of sperm preparation.

In this chapter the following aspects are discussed:

(1) Technical aspects of IUI;

(2) Ovarian stimulation for IUI.

TECHNICAL ASPECTS

Technical aspects that might influence the outcome of IUI are sperm preparation techniques and the technique of IUI itself.

Sperm preparation techniques

Although sperm preparation techniques are predominantly used in ART, such as IVF or ICSI, for IUI sperm must also be prepared, and for this reason an overview of the different methodologies is given.

The aim of sperm preparation is to provide as many normal, motile sperm as possible in order to increase the chances of fertilizing the oocyte *in vitro* (IVF or ICSI) or *in vivo* (IUI). Furthermore, motile sperm should be separated from seminal plasma containing debris, dead cells, etc.

For all sperm preparation techniques it has to be considered that damage to the sperm from dilution, temperature change, centrifugation and exposure to potentially toxic material must be minimized. Dilutions should be done slowly, especially with cryopreserved sperm. Temperature changes should be gradual. Preparation of the insemination suspension should be performed at 37°C. Centrifugal force should be the lowest possible required to bring down the sperm cells. Minimizing centrifugation, particularly in the absence of seminal plasma, and separating the live motile sperm from the dead sperm and debris early in the procedure should limit oxidative damage caused by free oxygen radicals released from leukocytes or abnormal sperm.

Methods

Numerous different techniques have been described for sperm preparation. Conservative infertility treatment including IUI usually uses relatively simple preparation techniques. The following section addresses only the three most common techniques. For more detailed information specialized literature should be referred to, such as the WHO Laboratory Manual for the Examination of Human Semen and Sperm–cervical Mucus Interaction[1].

Sperm washing

Sperm washing can be considered as the simplest sperm preparation technique. It involves repeated washing of the sperm by dilution of the semen with culture medium supplemented with protein, followed by centrifugation and resuspension of the pellet. The yield of motile sperm cells is usually lower compared with other methods. However, for laboratories performing only IUI it might be acceptable, as they usually handle samples with reletively normal sperm parameters and therefore the yield of motile sperm is not as crucial as for other ART procedures.

Swim-up

The swim-up preparation technique has been described in several different ways. The seminal plasma is usually overlaid directly with culture medium. This allows the sperm to swim from the seminal plasma into the culture medium. The upper layer can then be removed and contains a relatively high concentration of motile sperm. Alternatively, the semen sample may be

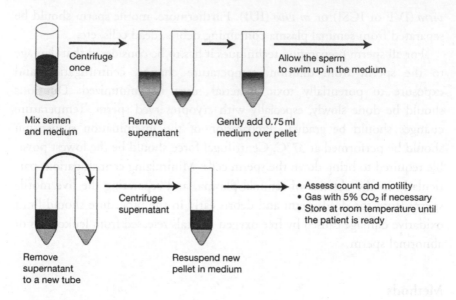

Figure 6.1   Pellet and swim-up technique

diluted and centrifuged and the pellet loosened and overlaid with culture medium again (Figure 6.1).

Density gradients

A variety of density gradient separation procedures have been described. The principal difference between these methods and the swim-up preparation is that they are quicker and easier to perform. The underlying principle for these techniques is that intact versus abnormal sperm reveal a different density and thereby may be separated by density gradients. Usually discontinuous gradients of two or more layers are used. The sperm samples are loaded on top of the gradients and undergo centrifugation. Motile sperm form a distinct band and can thereby be isolated (Figure 6.2). Overall the recovery of sperm is greater with the gradient techniques compared with the swim-up technique. However, the progressive motility is usually lower.

A recent review of trials on different semen preparation techniques for IUI was published by Boomsma et al.[2]. In this review the authors compared sperm washing versus swim-up technique versus density gradients. If semen parameters after preparation were analyzed as an endpoint there seemed to be an advantage for gradient techniques. However, there was no statistically

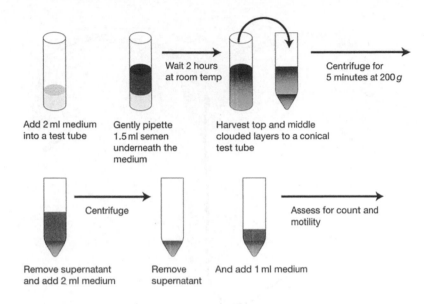

Wait 2 hours at room temp

Centrifuge for 5 minutes at 200 g

Add 2 ml medium into a test tube

Gently pipette 1.5 ml semen underneath the medium

Harvest top and middle clouded layers to a conical test tube

Centrifuge

Assess for count and motility

Remove supernatant and add 2 ml medium

Remove supernatant

And add 1 ml medium

Figure 6.2 Standard swim-up or layering technique

significant difference between pregnancy rates for these three methods, and no significant difference in the miscarriage rate per couple or multiple pregnancy rate was observed. The overall conclusion provided by the authors was that there was insufficient evidence to recommend any specific preparation technique, as sufficient data were not available.

The technique for IUI is relatively simple (Figure 6.3). Fresh semen samples should be available for preparation at least 2 hours prior to the IUI procedure, and the prepared sample kept at a temperature of 37°C prior to the insemination (see above). The procedure is carried out gently and atraumatically, using aseptic techniques.

The patient is usually placed in the lithotomy position. The cervix is exposed and if excessive cervical mucus is seen, the cervix is gently wiped with cotton balls soaked in warm sterile saline. Thereafter, the insemination catheter is attached to a 1-ml syringe, both are rinsed with warm culture medium and the sperm sample is loaded into the catheter at a volume of 0.3–1.0 ml. The catheter is gently passed through the cervical canal into the uterine cavity, and the semen sample is slowly expelled. Care should be taken not to touch the fundus with the catheter, because this might cause uterine contractions, which are thought to influence negatively the outcome of the procedure. Thus it is an advantage if the length of the

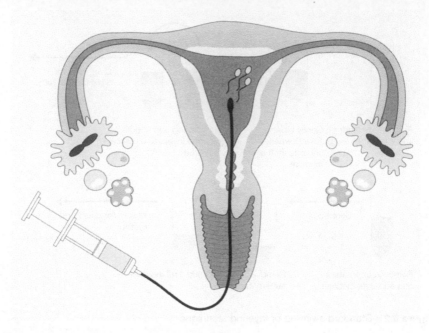

Figure 6.3   Intrauterine insemination technique

uterine cavity of the patient has been determined at a previous ultrasound examination.

Single versus double IUI

There has been much debate as to whether double IUI in one treatment cycle might increase pregnancy rates. In a recent publication based on a Cochrane Review, Cantineau *et al.*[3] analyzed three studies involving 386 patients. Although the results showed a pregnancy rate per cycle in favor of double insemination, there was no significant effect of double insemination on pregnancy rate per couple. The authors concluded that, based on the results of two trials, double IUI showed no significant benefit over single IUI in the treatment of subfertile couples.

OVARIAN STIMULATION FOR IUI

In order to understand the principles of ovarian stimulation for IUI the following aspects should be considered:

- The aim of controlled ovarian hyperstimulation (COH) in ART cycles (IVF/ICSI) is to retrieve a sufficiently high number of good-quality oocytes in order to achieve a pregnancy

- The aim of ovulation induction in anovulatory patients (e.g. those with polycystic ovary syndrome (PCOS)) is to achieve monofollicular development and ovulation of a single follicle to induce a spontaneous pregnancy

- The aim of mild ovarian hyperstimulation (MOH) for IUI is to support mono/oligofollicular development in women who usually ovulate, in order to increase the chance for a pregnancy and at the same time control the risk for multiple gestation. In clinical practice this means that most clinicians would cancel an IUI cycle if more than three mature follicles are detected after MOH and they would carefully counsel the patient about the risk of multiple pregnancies when 2–3 follicles are detected

Before different protocols for MOH in IUI are discussed, it is important to understand that several factors influence the individual patient's response to ovarian stimulation. We can differentiate patient-related (endogenous) factors, which – in most cases – cannot be influenced by the physician, and treatment-related (exogenous) factors, which refer to the treatment protocol used and the drugs applied for ovarian stimulation. These issues will be discussed below.

Factors influencing ovarian response

Ovarian stimulation is a key element of different types of infertility treatment[4]. Especially for ART the number and quality of oocytes retrieved are determinants of success; even though a high number of oocytes does not necessarily predict a good outcome[5], it has been shown that the number of fertilized oocytes achieved directly correlates with the chance of achieving a pregnancy[6]. However, not only for ART but also for ovulation induction and COH prior to IUI the ovarian response is an important predictive factor.

Several predictive factors such as age, antral follicle count, day-3 follicle stimulating hormone (FSH) levels, inhibin B, anti-Müllerian hormone, etc. have been shown to correlate with a patient's individual outcome of a treatment cycle. Furthermore, genetic factors such as FSH receptor genotype[7] or estrogen receptor polymorphism help to classify a patient as a low, normal or high responder and hence adapt the dose for gonadotropin treatment accordingly. Genetic variations in the metabolism of clomiphene have been described to explain the different response rates to this drug[8]. Obviously, these patient-related factors cannot be changed in order to influence an ovarian response. However, in addition to patient-related factors, the choice of a specific drug for ovarian stimulation might influence the ovarian response.

In women with adequate ovarian reserve, response to stimulation treatment varies only within a certain range. In these women it has been shown that antral follicle count may be used as a predictor of ovarian response, as this determines the number of follicles that will grow in response to gonadotropin stimulation in that particular cycle[9].

However, in patients with diminished ovarian reserve, there seems to be much more variability in response to gonadotropin stimulation, due to the higher variability of antral follicles available.

The varying number of antral follicles available is reflected by the change of FSH levels from cycle to cycle in these patients. This also explains why measuring FSH in two consecutive spontaneous cycles may predict the remaining ovarian reserve better than with a single measurement[10]. However, even with two measurements a substantial number of patients are still misdiagnosed with regard to their ovarian responsiveness.

Repetitive stimulation procedures and cycle-to-cycle variability

Patients undergoing repetitive cycles of ovarian stimulation for IVF/ICSI did not demonstrate a decrease in the number of oocytes produced. This was confirmed by the limited variations in consecutive cycles for IUI treatment of regularly menstruating and ovulating patients. The OMEGA project group, which is an ongoing prospective cohort study in The Netherlands, could not demonstrate a decrease in the number of oocytes retrieved in those patients who underwent at least seven consecutive IVF cycles, from cycle 1 to cycle 6 after adjusting for the patient's age. Similar observations have been published by other workers[11].

Caligara et al. studied oocyte donors and could not see any impairment of oocyte number or quality in consecutive cycles. However, it should be noted that oocyte donors would not have pre-existing impairment of ovarian function compared with infertile patients[12]. Therefore, if ovarian function is already impaired before stimulation therapy, a decrease in the number of oocytes retrieved may occur, as was shown in patients with ovarian endometriomas[13].

In conclusion, in patients with intact ovarian reserve, repetitive high-dose ovarian stimulation does not increase the risk of higher cycle-to-cycle variability, but in patients with impaired ovarian function it might decrease the number of oocytes retrieved after consecutive stimulation cycles. The number of oocytes retrieved is usually chosen as the primary endpoint to look at cycle-to-cycle variability, as the majority of studies published to date are lacking statistical power to look at clinical pregnancy rate or even live birth rate. Nonetheless, these would be the most relevant endpoints to consider to investigate whether cycle-to-cycle variability is just a phenomenon that might be observed during ovarian stimulation without any clinical relevance, or whether this has an impact on the overall outcome of IUI or ART treatment.

CYCLE-TO-CYCLE VARIABILITY IN DIFFERENT STIMULATION REGIMENS

Clomiphene citrate

There are no data available on the cycle-to-cycle variability in the response to clomiphene citrate (CC). However, differences in metabolism and individual receptor distribution – i.e. the genetic disposition of the patient – may play a role in the individual response of the endometrium as well as the pituitary release of FSH to stimulate the ovary endogenously.

Since body mass index (BMI), severity of oligo/amenorrhea and grade of hyperandrogenemia are predictors of the ovarian response to CC in PCOS patients, the biological variations of these parameters, especially hyperandrogenemia, may influence the response to the drug.

The variation of the ovarian response to different doses of CC or from cycle-to-cycle may be small, since overall the number of stimulated follicles does not vary widely when 50 mg CC is compared with 100 mg or 150 mg for 5 days. This is reflected in the relatively low risk of multiple pregnancies with CC treatment (about 10–15%) even if high-order multiple gestations are possible. This leads some authors to suggest monitoring only the first cycle with a certain dose, since cycle-to-cycle variation seems to be small[14].

OVULATION INDUCTION WITH LOW-DOSE GONADOTROPINS

Low-dose ovarian stimulation, especially in WHO group II patients suffering from PCOS, has been evaluated extensively. It is recommended, however, that in a step-up protocol the last dose used should be chosen as the initial dose in a new treatment cycle with the step-down protocol after cancellation of the stimulation cycle for no response of follicular growth[15]. This reflects the experience of an apparently relatively constant dose response from cycle to cycle.

Van Santbrink et al.[16] described a group of 56 patients who had been treated for ovulation induction with a step-down protocol. In 25% of patients the dose was changed initially from the standard of 150 IU daily to either a higher or a lower starting dose for the subsequent cycle – based on experience with previous stimulation cycles. The authors observed three groups of patients during the treatment cycle: those who had an early step down of the human menopausal gonadotropin (hMG) dose (group A), those with the standard procedure (group B) and those with a dose increase or no change of the initial dose (group C). Interestingly, those in group A had a mean of 28.5 IU above the predicted effective starting dose, those in group B a mean of 13 IU above the predicted dose and those in group C a mean of 43 IU under the predicted starting dose in the subsequent cycle. This prediction was made using a previously established model[17]. The authors argued, that cycle-to-cycle variation occurs only in a small range[16]. However, they also agreed that this hypothesis has to be proven in future studies.

PROTOCOLS FOR OVARIAN STIMULATION PRIOR TO IUI

As indicated above, the rationale to use MOH in conjunction with IUI is that it improves timing, corrects subtle cycle disorders and at the same time increases the number of available oocytes[18]. Furthermore most authors would now agree that IUI in combination with stimulated cycles is more effective than IUI without stimulation. However, as at the same time risks for multiple pregnancies and ovarian hyperstimulation syndrome (OHSS) are increased, MOH should only be applied if it is proven to be effective and if careful monitoring is guaranteed.

Recent studies indicate that the efficacy of MOH in IUI clearly depends on the indication for the procedure:

- For patients with 'cervical factor' the benefit of MOH has never been demonstrated in a large randomized controlled trial

- For patients with male factor infertility the benefit of MOH seems to depend on the degree of male infertility: in case of a 'mild male factor' MOH seems to increase conception rates, whereas in 'severe male factor' infertility the benefit of MOH could not be shown. Obviously the crucial question is how to define mild and severe male factor properly

- For patients with unexplained (idiopathic) infertility MOH seems to increase pregnancy rates

In summary, according to current knowledge MOH improves the outcome of IUI in patients with mild male factor infertility as well as in patients with idiopathic infertility, whereas its benefits have not been shown in patients with cervical factor, or severe male factor infertility.

For MOH, different drugs are available. Today, CC can still be seen as the 'gold standard' in terms of first-line treatment, especially for chronic anovulatory patients, and it is widely used because it is cheap, easy to apply and regarded as being effective. Usually CC is given at doses between 50 mg and 150 mg for 5–6 days (e.g. cycle days 5–9). The mechanism of action is described in Chapter 5.1 of this book.

Approximately 30–40% of patients show CC resistance. Although there is no consensus on a clear definition of CC resistance, most clinicians would consider a patient CC resistant if, in three consecutive cycles and in spite of dose increase, follicular development/ovulation could not be achieved. For CC-resistant patients gonadotropins are usually given as second-line treatment. Although they have been proved effective in these patients, gonadotropin treatment regimens require subcutaneous injections and are more expensive compared with CC regimens. Therefore, a careful risk–benefit analysis needs to be performed defining first- and second-line MOH treatment for IUI.

As in many other fields, results from randomized trials comparing the effects of two different drugs are contradictory. Whereas Balasch et al.[19] and Matorras et al.[20] showed superiority of low-dose FSH treatment compared with CC for IUI, Ecochard et al.[21] did not demonstrate any significant difference between CC and gonadotropin treatment. Karlström et al.[22]

published a trial in which eight different treatment regimens were compared and came to the conclusion that, for IUI, gonadotropin treatment was more effective than CC treatment. This was confirmed by Guzick et al.[23] who analyzed 45 trials and showed that IUI plus gonadotropins (pregnancy rate 18% per cycle) was more effective than IUI plus CC (6.7% pregnancy rate per cycle) and IUI in a natural cycle (4% pregnancy rate per cycle).

On the basis of these data the conclusion can be drawn that MOH for IUI using gonadotropins is more effective than CC[18]. Compared with CC treatment, gonadotropin treatment can be seen as more 'aggressive' as it has been shown that pregnancy rates increase with increasing dose of gonadotropins. However, at the same time multiple pregnancy rates also increase. Therefore, careful monitoring of gonadotropin therapy is mandatory.

The most important parameter for monitoring of gonadotropin treatment is the number and size of follicles developing under treatment. In addition to follicular size, estradiol levels can be used as predictive factors for multifollicular development and, thus, for the risk of multiple gestation. From the studies published to date it is impossible to agree on a concrete critical upper threshold for estradiol levels; however, it is obvious that the probability of achieving a multiple pregnancy is correlated with the aggressiveness of the stimulation protocol and at the same time it is correlated with the criteria that are applied for cycle cancellation. The more strictly these criteria are defined, the lower the risk for multiple gestation, and if more risk is taken during stimulation and monitoring, the risk for multiple gestation increases.

Guzick et al.[24] showed, in a randomized controlled trial, that IUI with MOH using gonadotropins in 231 couples achieved a higher pregnancy rate (33%) compared with natural cycles in 234 couples (18%). However, there was no multiple pregnancy in the group of 42 couples achieving a pregnancy in the natural cycle, whereas 22 multiple pregnancies occurred in the group of 77 pregnancies in the gonadotropin group. The type of gonadotropin stimulation applied in this trial should be noted, as it is striking that gonadotropins were started at a dose of 150 IU from day 3–7 of the cycle. This can be seen as a relatively high dose for an IUI regimen, because most of the young patients in IVF/ICSI cycles would be put on this starting dose. Goverde et al.[25] showed that the risk for multiple pregnancies could be properly controled in IUI cycles if a low-dose protocol was applied and strict criteria were established for canceling the cycles. In their study the authors canceled the cycle if more than three follicles of > 17 mm were detected or there were six follicles of > 13 mm.

REFERENCES

1. World Health Organization. Laboratory Manual for the Examination of Human Semen and Sperm–cervical Mucus Interaction, 4th edn. New York: Cambridge University Press, 1999

2. Boomsma CM, Heineman MJ, Cohlen BJ, Farquhar C. Semen preparation techniques for intrauterine insemination. Cochrane Database Syst Rev 2004; (3): CD004507

3. Cantineau AE, Heineman MJ, Cohlen BJ. Single versus double intrauterine insemination in stimulated cycles for subfertile couples: a systematic review based on a Cochrane review. Hum Reprod 2003; 18: 941–6

4. Keck C, Bassett R, Ludwig M. Factors influencing response to ovarian stimulation. RBM Online 2005; 5: 562–9

5. Inge GB, Brinsden PR, Elder KT. Oocyte number per live birth in IVF: were Steptoe and Edwards less wasteful? Hum Reprod 2005; 20: 588–92

6. Templeton A. Avoiding multiple pregnancies in ART: replace as many embryos as you like – one at a time. Hum Reprod 2000; 15; 1662

7. Greb RR, Behre HM, Simoni M. Pharmacogenetics in ovarian stimulation – current concepts and future options. Reprod Biomed Online 2005; 11: 589–600

8. Rostami-Hodjegan A, Lennard MS, Tucker GT, Ledger WR. Monitoring plasma concentrations to individualize treatment with clomiphene citrate. Fertil Steril 2004; 81: 1187–93

9. Hendriks DJ, Mol BW, Bancsi LF, et al. Antral follicle count in the prediction of poor ovarian response and pregnancy after in vitro fertilization: a meta-analysis and comparison with basal follicle-stimulating hormone level. Fertil Steril 2005; 83: 291–301

10. Bancsi LF, Broekmans FJ, Looman CW, et al. Predicting poor ovarian response in IVF: use of repeat basal FSH measurement. J Reprod Med 2004; 49: 187–94

11. Schroder AK, Katalinic A, Diedrich K, Ludwig M. Cumulative pregnancy rates and drop-out rates in a German IVF programme: 4102 cycles in 2130 patients. Reprod Biomed Online 2004; 8: 600–6

12. Caligara C, Navarro J, Vargas G, et al. The effect of repeated controlled ovarian stimulation in donors. Hum Reprod 2001; 16: 2320–3

13. Al Azemi M, Bernal AL, Steele J, et al. Ovarian response to repeated controlled stimulation in in-vitro fertilization cycles in patients with ovarian endometriosis. Hum Reprod 2000; 15: 72–5

14. Nasseri S, Ledger WL. Clomiphene citrate in the twenty-first century. Hum Fertil 2001; 4: 145–51

15. Mulders AG, Eijkemans MJ, Imani B, Fauser BC. Prediction of chances for success or complications in gonadotrophin ovulation induction in normogonadotrophic anovulatory infertility. Reprod Biomed Online 2003; 7: 170–8

16. Van Santbrink EJ, Eijkemans MJ, Macklon NS, Fauser BC. FSH response-dose can be predicted in ovulation induction for normogonadotropic anovulatory infertility. Eur J Endocrinol 2002; 147: 223–6

17. Imani B, Eijkemans MJ, Faessen GH, et al. Prediction of the individual follicle-stimulating hormone threshold for gonadotrophin induction of ovulation in normogonadotropic anovulatory infertility: an approach to increase safety and efficiency. Fertil Steril 2002; 77: 83–90

18. Cohlen BJ. Should we continue performing intrauterine inseminations in the year 2004? Gynecol Obstet Invest 2005; 59: 3–13

19. Balasch J, Penarrubia J, Ballesca JL, et al. Intrauterine insemination, cervical pregnancy and successful treatment with methotrexate. Hum Reprod 1994; 9: 1580–3

20. Matorras R, Diaz T, Corcostegui B, et al. Ovarian stimulation in intrauterine insemination with donor sperm: a randomized prospective study comparing clomiphene citrate in fixed protocol versus highly purified urinary FSH. Hum Reprod 2002; 17: 2107–11
21. Ecochard R, Mathieu C, Royere D, et al. A randomized prospective study comparing pregnancy rates after clomiphene citrate and human menopausal gonadotropin before intrauterine insemination. Fertil Steril 2000; 73: 90–3
22. Karlström PO, Bergh T, Lundkvist O. A prospective randomized trial of artificial insemination versus intercourse in cycles stimulated with human menopausal gonadotropin or clomiphene citrate. Fertil Steril 1993; 59: 554–9
23. Guzick DS, Sullivan MW, Adamson GD, et al. Efficacy of treatment for unexplained infertility. Fertil Steril 1998; 70: 207–13
24. Guzick DS, Carson SA, Coutifaris C, et al. Efficacy of superovulation and intrauterine insemination in the treatment of infertility. National Cooperative Reproductive Medicine Network. N Engl J Med 1999; 340: 177–83
25. Goverde AJ, McDonnell J, Vermeiden JP, et al. Intrauterine insemination or in-vitro fertilisation in idiopathic subfertility and male subfertility: a randomized trial and cost-effectiveness analysis. Lancet 2000; 355: 13–18

7

Recurrent miscarriages

ETIOLOGY

In order to be able to discuss the topic of recurrent miscarriage and to interpret literature published on this topic, clinical versus biochemical pregnancies and early versus late miscarriages have to be clearly differentiated.

Studies indicate that the majority of biochemical pregnancies, i.e. subclinical pregnancies with a positive serum or urine concentration of human chorionic gonadotropin (hCG), are aborted spontaneously[1]. Clinically recognized pregnancies, i.e. those diagnosed with transvaginal ultrasonography, will end in a miscarriage in approximately 15–20% of cases and thus usually remain a single event in a woman's reproductive life. Recurrent miscarriage (RM), defined as three or more consecutive pregnancy losses before 20 weeks' gestation, affects 0.5–1% of women[2]. Most women with RM have recurrent pre-embryonic or embryonic losses. Recurrent fetal loss is less common, and recurrent fetal loss at or beyond 14 weeks of gestation is infrequent. Whether RM represents the common endpoint of independent etiological factors or a distinct pathophysiological entity, is unknown.

A wide variety of RM-associated pathologies have been identified, among them uterine anomalies[3], luteal phase defect[4], hyperprolactinemia[5], hyperandrogenemia[6], hyperhomocysteinuria[7] and genital infections[8].

Investigators found that 36–56% of women with recurrent pregnancy loss have polycystic ovary syndrome (PCOS) diagnosed by ultrasound examination of the ovaries[5]. However, ultrasonographic evidence of PCOS in women with RM does not predict a worse pregnancy outcome than in women with recurrent pregnancy loss without PCOS. Abortion rates of women with PCOS have been described to decline after laparoscopic ovarian drilling and after therapy with insulin sensitizers such as metformin. This adds credibility to the claim that high serum levels of androgens and/or luteinizing hormone (LH) increases the risk of miscarriage.

Genetic factors also contribute to RM. Maternal and paternal balanced translocations are found in 2–5% of couples with RM[9]. Familial clustering of recurrent miscarriage has also been described, suggesting an inherited component for this condition. In this respect, skewed inactivation of X chromosome and human leukocyte antigen (HLA) haplotype sharing have been advocated as etiological genetic factors of recurrent miscarriage. Moreover, single gene defects, e.g. mutations and polymorphisms, have been associated with RM. For example, a role for the HLA system[10], the pathway of folic acid metabolism[11] and the blood clotting cascade have been described[12].

A genetic or biochemical thrombophilic disposition seems to exert an etiological role in spontaneous abortion as well as RM. It has been suggested that thrombosis formation in the placenta in women with thrombophilia reduces placental perfusion, thus compromising the oxygen and nutrition supply to the fetus. In a meta-analysis of 31 studies, Rey et al. concluded that various thrombophilic factors were significantly associated with early and late spontaneous miscarriage as well as RM[13]. Specifically, they found that carriage of the factor V Leiden mutation was associated with early (odds ratio (OR) 2.01, 95% confidence interval (CI) 1.13, 3.58) and late (OR 7.83, 95% CI 2.83, 21.67) recurrent fetal loss, and late non-recurrent fetal loss (OR 3.26, 95% CI 1.82, 5.83). Activated protein C resistance was associated with early recurrent fetal loss (OR 3.48, 95% CI 1.58, 7.69), and prothrombin G20210A mutation with early recurrent (OR 2.56, 95% CI 1.04, 0.29) and late non-recurrent (OR 2.30, 95% CI 1.09, 4.87) fetal loss. Protein S deficiency was associated with recurrent fetal loss (OR 14.72, 95% CI 0.99, 218.01) and late non-recurrent fetal loss (OR 7.39, 95% CI 1.28, 42.63).

Despite a comprehensive diagnostic workup, however, a suspected cause will not be identified in up to 50% of cases. Immunological factors are believed to be involved in these cases of RM. Autoimmune dysfunctions, e.g. antiphospholipid syndrome, antithyroid autoantibodies, and anti-single-strand DNA autoantibodies, are found in 5–10% of affected women[14,15]. In addition, a growing body of evidence points to a central etiological role of alloimmune dysfunctions in women with idiopathic RM. Physiologically, the maternal immune system confronts the embryo/fetus with a host-defense reaction, based on the recognition of paternally derived fetal and placental antigens. To avoid rejection of the semiallogenic embryo/fetus, the maternal immune response is thoroughly suppressed in physiological pregnancies. A reduction of proinflammatory cytokines by the T helper cell TH-1/TH-2 balance shift[16], lymphatic production of progesterone-induced blocking factor (PIBF)[17], increased production of asymmetrically glycosylated blocking antibodies[18], and fetal shutdown of maternal T-cell proliferation by local tryptophan deficiency[19] are the most prominent mechanisms to guarantee embryonic/fetal evasion of the maternal immune attack.

This fetal defense system seems to be impaired in women with RM. Lower serum levels of asymmetrically glycosylated antibodies have been described among affected women[18]. Moreover, a lack of the physiological TH-1/TH-2 balance shift and elevated serum levels of proinflammatory cytokines have been found among women with recurrent miscarriage[20].

In summary, various factors seem to be associated with RM. Most of these factors, however, have not been proven to be causally linked to RM. Most investigators consider only the following to be etiological factors of RM:

- Maternal/paternal chromosome anomalies

- The antiphospholipid syndrome

- Genetically or biochemically proven thrombophilia

- Presence of a uterine septum

DIAGNOSTIC PROCEDURES

Although RM has been defined as three consecutive spontaneous abortions, the risk of abortion after two successive abortions (30%) is clinically similar to the risk of recurrence among women with three or more consecutive abortions (33%)[21]. Thus, patients with two or more consecutive spontaneous abortions are candidates for an evaluation to determine the etiology, if any, for their pregnancy losses.

Based on the assumption that the presence of a uterine septum, abnormal maternal and/or paternal karyotype, antiphospholipid syndrome, or genetic and/or biochemical thrombophilia are etiological factors of RM, appropriate diagnostic procedures should be performed.

Parental karyotype

Parental cytogenetic analysis should be offered to all couples with RM. In addition, all couples diagnosed with a balanced translocation or inversion should be offered prenatal genetic diagnosis because of the increased risk of a karyotypic abnormality in the conceptus.

It is not necessary to obtain a karyotype of the aborted fetus/tissue except for scientific purposes. Studies to date have not convincingly demonstrated that an aneuploid fetal karyotype rules out a maternal cause or alters the treatment of the affected couple. Also, the prognostic value of the fetal karyotype has been discussed controversially and no evidence-based recommendation can be given in this respect.

Uterine anomalies

An exploration of the uterine cavity is recommended in women with RM. Although this can be done by hysterosalpingography, three-dimensional transvaginal ultrasonography and sonohysterography, we recommend performing a hysteroscopy with local anesthesia on an outpatient basis. It has been demonstrated that this method is feasible, efficient and well accepted by patients[22]. We use rigid endoscopes, which have been shown to be superior to flexible endoscopes for outpatient hysteroscopy[23].

Antiphospholipid syndrome

Women with RM should be tested for the presence of antiphospholipid syndrome, which can be expected in up to 15% of cases. Antiphospholipid syndrome is identified by the presence of RM and/or thrombosis and the detection of lupus anticoagulant, β_2-glycoprotein I-dependent anticardiolipin antibodies, or both on two occasions at least 6 weeks apart[24]. The IgG isotype of anticardiolipin is clinically most relevant, but tests repeatedly positive for IgM anticardiolipin are also sufficient to establish the diagnosis.

Thrombophilia

Tests for the factor V Leiden mutation, the prothrombin G20210A mutation and deficiencies of protein C, protein S and antithrombin III should be performed.

TREATMENT

Although many clinicians treat women with RM and thrombophilia with heparin, it has to be acknowledged that there is only weak evidence supporting this treatment. No randomized controlled trial has proved heparin to be an effective therapy in women with RM and thrombophilia. There are, however, retrospective studies and prospective, uncontrolled trials claiming that abortion rates in these women are significantly lower when using low-molecular-weight heparin[25,26]. Two randomized studies with 242 participants investigated subgroups of women with RM. In one study, 54 pregnant women with RM without detectable anticardiolipin antibodies were randomized to low-dose aspirin or placebo. Similar live-birth rates were observed in both groups (relative risk (RR) 1.00, 95% CI 0.78, 1.29). In another study, a subgroup of 20 women who had had a previous fetal loss after the 20th week and had a thrombophilic defect were randomized to enoxaparin or aspirin. Enoxaparin treatment resulted in an increased live-birth rate as compared with low-dose aspirin (RR 10.00, 95% CI 1.56, 64.20). A Cochrane review on this subject concluded that the evidence on the efficacy and safety of thromboprophylaxis with aspirin and heparin in women with a history of at least two spontaneous miscarriages or one late intrauterine fetal death without apparent causes other than inherited thrombophilia was too limited to recommend the use of anticoagulants outside of clinical trials[27].

No randomized clinical trial has established corticosteroids as effective therapy of women with RM. Published randomized trials demonstrated no significant effect and the available retrospective studies on this issue produced controversial results[21].

If a uterine septum is diagnosed, it should be removed by hysteroscopic resection, shown to be a safe outpatient method[21]. No controlled trial, however, has shown that the correction of uterine anatomic abnormalities positively influenced the outcome of the next pregnancy. Retrospectively analyzed case series suggest that 70–85% of women with RM with a uterine septum who undergo surgical correction will deliver liveborn infants in their next pregnancies[28], but these excellent results are subject to criticism.

In women with RM and the antiphospholipid syndrome, a combination therapy with aspirin and heparin should be initiated. The efficacy of this treatment has been demonstrated in prospective randomized trials. Two studies have shown that women with RM and positive test results for antiphospholipid antibodies benefited from treatment with low-dose aspirin and heparin with successful pregnancy rates between 70 and 75%, compared with less than 50% for the untreated patients[29,30]. These studies used heparin dosages in the range of 10 000–25 000 U per day.

Immunotherapies have been tested for their efficacy in women with RM. The most widely used immunotherapeutic treatment regimen for women with RM involves immunizing the female partner with the male partner's leukocytes. Randomized trials and meta-analyses of these trials, however, have demonstrated no significant effect of this treatment[21]. In addition, there is no consensus regarding patient selection and treatment schemes, and these therapies carry a risk of viral transmission and triggering of autoimmune disease. In summary, immunization techniques should not be used outside of clinical trials.

The second immunomodulatory therapy used as a treatment for RM involves intravenous infusions of immunoglobulins (IVIG). It has been suggested that IVIG contains antibodies that block antibody-mediated immune damage and induces T-cell receptor blockade, inhibition of natural killer (NK)-cell activity, inhibition of TH-1 cytokine secretion, Fc-receptor blockade, complement inactivation, down-regulation of B-cell responsiveness and enhanced T-cell suppressor function. However, randomized trials and two meta-analyses of these randomized trials failed to demonstrate a clear clinical benefit of this treatment[31,32].

Progesterone may improve the outcome of women with RM. We recommend using progesterone supplementation in early pregnancy, based on the results of a meta-analysis of three randomized trials[4]. The resulting OR for pregnancies reaching at least 20 weeks' gestation was 3.09 (95% CI 1.28, 7.42), which indicates that progesterone given in early pregnancy is useful in women with RM. Also, a Cochrane review found that, in a subgroup analysis of three trials involving women with RM, progestogen treatment showed a statistically significant decrease of the miscarriage rate compared with placebo or no treatment (OR 0.39, 95% CI 0.17, 0.91)[33]. Progesterone may be given orally, intravaginally, or intramuscularly. There is no clear recommendation as to the superiority of a specific route of application in women with RM. Based on data generated in *in vitro* fertilization (IVF) trials, it may be argued that intramuscular application of progesterone may be superior to the other routes, but it is associated with more discomfort to the patient.

In accordance with recommendations for healthy women, women with RM should supplement folate 400 µg/day before conception and up to 15 weeks of gestation.

In summary, the following treatments are recommended:

- Uterine septum dissection if present

- Oral/intravaginal/intramuscularly progesterone supplementation up to 15 weeks' gestation

- Low-molecular-weight heparin in women with RM and thrombophilia

- Aspirin 100 mg/day and heparin 10 000–25 000 U/day in women with RM and antiphospholipid syndrome

The following treatments are not recommended outside of clinical trials:

- Paternal leukocyte immunization

- IVIG

- Corticosteroids

REFERENCES

1. Boklage CE. Survival probability of human conceptions from fertilization to term. Int J Fertil 1990; 35: 75–94
2. Wilcox AJ, Weinberg CR, O'Connor JF. Incidence of early loss of pregnancy. N Engl J Med 1988; 319: 189–94
3. Tho PT, Byrd JR, McDonough PG. Etiologies and subsequent reproductive performance of 100 couples with recurrent abortion. Fertil Steril 1979; 32: 389–95
4. Daya S. Efficacy of progesterone support for pregnancy in women with recurrent miscarriage. A meta-analysis of controlled trials. Br J Obstet Gynaecol 1989; 96: 275–80
5. Kutteh WH. Recurrent pregnancy loss: an update. Curr Opin Obstet Gynecol 1999; 11: 435–9
6. Okon MA, Laird SM, Tuckerman EM. Serum androgen levels in women who have recurrent miscarriages and their correlation with markers of endometrial function. Fertil Steril 69: 682–90
7. Wouters MG, Boers GH, Blom HJ, et al. (Hyperhomocysteinemia: a risk factor in women with unexplained recurrent early pregnancy loss. Fertil Steril 1998; 60: 820–5
8. Witkin SS, Ledger, WJ. Antibodies to Chlamydia trachomatis in sera of women with recurrent spontaneous abortions. Am J Obstet Gynecol 1992; 67: 135–9
9. Husslein P, Huber J, Wagenbichler P. Chromsome abnormalities in 150 couples with multiple spontaneous abortions. Fertil Steril 1982; 37: 379–83
10. Takakuwa K, Hataya I, Arakawa M. Possible susceptibility of the HLA-DPB1*0402 and HLA-DPB1*04 alleles to unexplained recurrent abortion: analysis by means of polymerase chain reaction-restricted fragment length polymorphism method. Am J Reprod Immunol 1992; 42: 233–9

11. Ray JG, Laskin CA. Folic acid and homocyst(e)ine metabolic defects and the risk of placental abruption, pre-eclampsia and pregnancy loss: a systematic review. Placenta 1999; 20: 519–29

12. Souza SS, Ferriani RA, Pontes AG. Factor V Leiden and factor II G20210A mutations in patients with recurrent abortion. Hum Reprod 1999; 14: 2448–50

13. Rey E, Kahn SR, David M, Shrier I. Thrombophilic disorders and fetal loss: a meta-analysis. Lancet 2003; 361: 901–8

14. Sugi T, Katsunuma J, Izumi S, et al. Prevalence and heterogeneity of antiphosphatidylethanolamine antibodies in patients with recurrent early pregnancy losses. Fertil Steril 1999; 71: 1060–5

15. Wilson R, Ling H, MacLean MA, et al. Thyroid antibody titer and avidity in patients with recurrent miscarriage. Fertil Steril 1999; 71: 558–61

16. Raghubathy R, Makhseed M, Azizieh F, et al. Maternal TH1-and TH2-type reactivity to placental antigens in normal human pregnancy and unexplained recurrent spontaneous abortions. Cell Immunol 1999; 196: 122–30

17. Szekeres-Bartho J, Wegmann TG. A progesterone-dependent immunomodulatory protein alters the TH1/TH2 balance. J Reprod Immunol 1996; 31: 81–95

18. Eblen AC, Gercel-Taylor C, Shields LB, et al. Alterations in humoral immune responses associated with recurrent pregnancy loss. Fertil Steril 2000; 2: 305–13

19. Munn DH, Zhou M, Attwood JT, et al. Prevention of allogeneic fetal rejection by tryptophan catabolism. Science 1998; 281: 1191–3

20. Jenkins C, Roberts J, Wilson R, et al. Evidence of a TH1 type response associated with recurrent miscarriage. Fertil Steril 2000; 6: 1206–12

21. American College of Obstetricians and Gynecologists. Management of recurrent early pregnancy loss. ACOG technical bulletin No. 24. Washington DC: American College of Obstetricians and Gynecologists, 2001

22. Wieser F, Kurz C, Wenzl R, et al. Atraumatic cervical passage at outpatient hysteroscopy. Fertil Steril 1998; 69: 549–51

23. Unfried G, Wieser F, Albrecht A, et al. Flexible versus rigid endoscopes for outpatient hysteroscopy: a prospective randomized clinical trial. Hum Reprod 2001; 16: 168–71

24. Yetman DL, Kutteh WH. Antiphospholipid antibody panels and recurrent pregnancy loss: prevalence of anticardiolipin antibodies compared with other antiphospholipid antibodies. Fertil Steril 1996; 66: 540–6

25. Brenner B, Bar J, Ellis M, et al; Live-Enox Investigators. Effects of enoxaparin on late pregnancy complications and neonatal outcome in women with recurrent pregnancy loss and thrombophilia: results from the Live-Enox study. Fertil Steril 2005; 84: 770–3

26. Glueck CJ, Wang P, Goldenberg N, Sieve L. Pregnancy loss, polycystic ovary syndrome, thrombophilia, hypofibrinolysis, enoxaparin, metformin. Clin Appl Thromb Hemost 2004; 10: 323–34

27. Di Nisio M, Peters L, Middeldorp S. Anticoagulants for the treatment of recurrent pregnancy loss in women without antiphospholipid syndrome. Cochrane Database Syst Rev 2005; (2): CD004734

28. March CM, Israel R. Hysteroscopic management of recurrent abortion caused by septate uterus. Am J Obstet Gynecol 1987; 156: 834–42

29. Kutteh WH. Antiphospholipid antibody-associated recurrent pregnancy loss: treatment with heparin and low-dose aspirin is superior to low-dose aspirin alone. Am J Obstet Gynecol 1996; 174: 1584–9

30. Rai R, Cohen H, Dave M, Regan L. Randomized controlled trial of aspirin and aspirin plus heparin in pregnant women with recurrent miscarriage associated with phospholipid antibodies (or antiphospholipid antibodies). Br Med J 1997; 314: 253–7

31. Daya S, Gunby J, Clark DA. Intravenous immunoglobulin therapy for recurrent spontaneous abortion: a meta-analysis. Am J Reprod Immunol 1998; 39: 69–76
32. Daya S, Gunby J, Porter F, et al. Critical analysis of intravenous immunoglobulin therapy for recurrent miscarriage. Hum Reprod Update 1999; 5: 475–82
33. Oates-Whitehead RM, Haas DM, Carrier JA. Progestogen for preventing miscarriage. Cochrane Database Syst Rev 2003; (4): CD003511

8

Risk management

OVARIAN HYPERSTIMULATION SYNDROME

Ovarian hyperstimulation syndrome (OHSS) is a potentially life-threatening complication of ovarian stimulation therapy. Severe forms complicate 0.5–1% of *in vitro* fertilization (IVF) cycles. Its cardinal features are marked ovarian enlargement and acute third-space fluid sequestration. The fluid shift from the intra- to the extravascular spaces in response to the increase in capillary permeability contributes most to the morbidity associated with OHSS[1]. Ascites, sometimes pleural and/or pericardial effusion, hypovolemia, oliguria and hydroelectrolytic disorders may develop in the course of OHSS. In the most severe cases, thromboembolic phenomena may occur as a result of hemoconcentration and coagulation disturbances.

Spontaneous forms of OHSS may occur, but these are very rare and always reported during pregnancy.

The pathophysiology of OHSS remains poorly understood, and there is no reliable test to predict which patients will develop severe OHSS. Human chorionic gonadotropin (hCG) is thought to play a crucial role in the development of the syndrome. The interaction between hCG and the follicle stimulating hormone (FSH) receptor could be an essential prerequisite in the development of spontaneous OHSS and could explain why symptoms in spontaneous cases of OHSS appear later than in iatrogenic OHSS, in which follicular recruitment and enlargement occur during the ovarian stimulation with exogenous FSH. Smits *et al.* described a mutation in the FSH receptor gene in a patient presenting spontaneous OHSS during each of her four pregnancies[2]. Also, hCG-induced angiogenesis seems to play an important

Table 8.1	OHSS classification. Modified from reference 3		
Grade	**Mild**	**Moderate**	**Severe**
1	Abdominal distension and discomfort		
2	Features of grade 1 plus nausea, vomiting and/or diarrhea; ovaries enlarged to 5–12 cm		
3		Features of mild OHSS plus ultrasonic evidence of ascites	
4			Features of moderate OHSS plus clinical evidence of ascites and/or hydrothorax or breathing difficulties
5			All of the above plus change in blood volume, increased blood viscosity due to hemoconcentration, coagulation abnormalities and diminished renal perfusion and function

etiological role in the development of OHSS. The data available so far support the notion that OHSS is a consequence of multiple corpora lutea formation associated with active angiogenesis and increased capillary permeability.

Several classifications have been proposed. The often used classification by Golan *et al.* is composed of five grades, based on a combination of clinical symptoms, signs, ultrasound findings and laboratory criteria. Table 8.1 shows the OHSS classification proposed by Golan *et al.* in 1989[3].

Typically, OHSS develops in weeks 3–5 of gestation. The signs and symptoms of severe OHSS consist of a distended abdomen with grossly enlarged ovaries, gastrointestinal discomfort and/or dyspnea. Severe OHSS (grade 5 of the Golan classification) can be complicated by hypovolemic shock, electrolyte disturbances, oliguria and/or thrombosis. Other complications of the syndrome are respiratory distress syndrome, adnexal torsion, vulvar edema, liver function abnormalities and hydroureter. Usually, OHSS is a self-limiting disorder. Death from OHSS is rare, but cases have been reported in the literature[4].

In a series of 165 patients with OHSS (101 singletons and 64 twins) and 156 IVF control patients (85 singletons and 71 twins), gestational diabetes mellitus (GDM) and pregnancy-induced hypertension (PIH) were evaluated and no differences were noted. In the OHSS group, GDM presented with an incidence of 9.9% for singletons and 9.4% for twins, and for the control group, 12.9% and 7.0%, respectively. PIH presented as 6.9% for singletons and 10.9% for twins in the OHSS group, and 8.2% and 7.0% for the control groups, respectively[5].

Lyons et al. were the first to describe two distinct patterns of OHSS: the early type that occurred 3–7 days after ovulation triggered by hCG, and the late type that occurred 12–17 days after hCG administration[6]. Late-onset OHSS may be more likely to be severe and is more likely to occur in multiple pregnancies.

Table 8.2 details management strategies in patients with OHSS according to Beerendonk et al.[7].

Severe OHSS can be almost totally prevented by withholding the ovulation-inducing trigger of hCG in patients at high risk, or by replacing hCG with gonadotropin releasing hormone (GnRH) agonist to trigger ovulation[8].

It has been proposed that, in normal and high-responder patients undergoing their first IVF attempt, it would be prudent to perform controlled ovarian stimulation (COS) with a GnRH antagonist in combination with a GnRH agonist to trigger ovulation. In patients in whom < 20 oocytes are retrieved, and in low responders (who are expected to recruit < 3–4 follicles) or patients ≥ 40 years old, the COS protocol should be individually tailored. If the combined GnRH antagonist/agonist or the tailored COS protocols yield ≥ 20 oocytes, the patient should be followed for 5 days after oocyte retrieval for signs of early OHSS (ultrasonographic signs of ascites, hematocrit levels for the degree of hemoconcentration). If signs develop, embryo transfer may be withheld and all resulting embryos cryopreserved[9]. This strategy, however, is controversial and its efficacy has not been convincingly proved in randomized trials.

A Cochrane review shows a clear benefit from administration of intravenous albumin at the time of oocyte retrieval in prevention of severe OHSS in high-risk cases. In absolute terms, for every 18 women at risk of severe OHSS, albumin infusion will save one more case[10]. According to data published by the Cochrane collaboration, there is insufficient evidence that embryo freezing or coasting, i.e. withholding of gonadotropins, significantly reduces the risk of OHSS.

Table 8.2   Management strategies in OHSS. Modified from reference 7

Classification	Clinical characteristics/ biochemical parameters	Management
A Mild	Abdominal distension Inconvenience	Accept as inevitable
B Moderate	A plus: Ascites on ultrasound Variable ovarian enlargement	Instruct patient carefully Self-monitoring of body weight Bedrest Abundant fluid intake Frequent follow-up (outpatient basis)
C Severe	B plus: Massive ascites Hypovolemia Hemoconcentration Oliguria Electrolyte imbalances	Hospitalization Consider paracentesis Intravenous fluid therapy (crystalloids/plasma expanders/albumin) Monitoring fluid balance Low-dose heparin prophylaxis Diuretics (only when hemodilution achieved) Correction of electrolytes
D Critical	C plus: Hct >55% Impaired renal perfusion Thromboembolism Impending multiorgan failure	C plus: Intensive care unit Continuous monitoring of hemodynamics Dopamine drip Perform paracentesis Intravenous heparin Consider termination of pregnancy

MULTIPLE PREGNANCIES

Women undergoing assisted reproduction have a higher risk of multiple pregnancies. The efforts to increase the success rates of infertility treatment have been accompanied by a rise in the rate of multifetal pregnancies. For example, almost half of all babies born after assisted reproduction in the USA and Europe are twins, and almost half of all twins result from infertility treatment[11,12]. Multiple pregnancies *per se* have a higher risk for maternal morbidity and fetal morbidity and mortality due to pregnancy complications, higher rates of intrapartum complications and cesarean section, and prematurity[13].

Singleton pregnancies after infertility treatment are associated with an elevated risk of prematurity, independent of the fact that infertile women being treated are significantly older than comparable fertile women. This is important to the extent that an ever increasing number of babies result from subfertility treatment and that these babies disproportionately contribute to the prematurity-related disease burden. Among singletons resulting from assisted reproduction, two meta-analyses showed a 5.3–6.2% excess rate of preterm birth (from 6.1% to 11.4% and from 5.3% to 11.5%), corresponding to an OR of 2.0[14,15].

These studies, however, also demonstrate that, in twin pregnancies, perinatal mortality is about 40% lower after assisted reproduction compared with natural conception. For example, Helmerhorst et al. reported that, in a systematic review of 25 controlled trials, relative risks for twins after assisted reproduction were 0.95 (0.78–1.15) for very preterm birth, 1.07 (1.02–1.13) for preterm birth, 0.89 (0.74–1.07) for very low birth weight, 1.03 (0.99–1.08) for low birth weight, 1.27 (0.97–1.65) for small for gestational age, 1.21 (1.11–1.32) for cesarean section, 1.05 (1.01–1.09) for admission to a neonatal intensive care unit and 0.58 (0.44–0.77) for perinatal mortality[14].

This issue, however, is controversial, since other large epidemiological studies showed that at least some subgroups of twins may have a worse prognosis after infertility treatment compared with naturally conceived twins. The adverse pregnancy outcome in twins after infertility treatment may be more pronounced in monozygotic and monochorionic twins, as indicated in a Danish study of 3438 (3393 liveborn) IVF/ICSI and 10 362 (10 239 liveborn) non-IVF/ICSI twins born between 1995 and 2000[16].

In a population-based study of 2915 naturally conceived and 1453 medically conceived twin pairs in Belgium, the dizygotic to monozygotic twinning ratio was 95.2 : 4.8 among medically conceived twins and 53.8 : 46.2 in the natural conception group ($p < 0.001$)[17]. In this study, medically conceived twins generally were more likely to be preterm delivered by cesarean section (odds ratio 1.5, 1.2–1.9). In particular, they observed an excess preterm birth rate of 11.7% in twins after IVF/intracytoplasmic sperm injection (ICSI), which is about twice the excess rate reported in singletons after IVF/ICSI compared with naturally conceived singletons.

Ovarian stimulation in the context of conservative infertility treatment using clomiphene citrate is associated with an increased risk of multiple pregnancy. Ovulation induction by ovarian stimulation outside of IVF/ICSI is estimated to be responsible for 20% of twin births and for 38% of triplet and higher-order multiple births. In absolute terms, the multiple livebirth rate after ovarian stimulation is between 2% and 13%[18]. Whether or not twins conceived after ovarian stimulation with clomiphene citrate have a worse outcome than naturally conceived twins, is unknown. In any case, the rate of multiple pregnancy with its inherent risks is increased compared with natural conceptions.

Singleton pregnancies after ovarian stimulation may have a slightly higher risk of miscarriage, but the perinatal outcome does not seem to be worse compared with natural conceptions. For example, in a prospective study of reproductive outcomes of 1744 clomiphene pregnancies and 3245 spontaneous pregnancies, the overall incidence of abortion was higher for clomiphene pregnancies (23.7% vs. 20.4%; $p < 0.01$)[19].

Clomiphene citrate has no teratogenic effect. In a series of 1034 pregnancies after clomiphene-induced ovulation and 30 033 babies after natural conception, no difference was identified. After clomiphene treatment, 14.2% of pregnancies ended in abortion, 0.5% in ectopic pregnancy, 0.1% in molar pregnancy and 1.6% in stillbirth. In all, 935 infants were born, and 21 (2.3%) showed visible malformations. This incidence of malformations was not significantly different from that among babies after spontaneous ovulation (1.7%), and the types of malformation after clomiphene treatment were similar to those of natural conception[20].

Recommendations to prevent multiple pregnancies caused by ovarian stimulation include withholding hCG administration when more than six follicles are ≥ 12 mm in diameter, when more than three follicles are ≥ 14 mm or ≥ 16 mm in diameter, when more than two or three follicles are ≥ 18 mm in diameter; and when estradiol concentration exceeds 400 pg/ml, 600 pg/ml, 1000 pg/ml, or 2000 pg/ml, depending on the study[21].

Also, it has been suggested that multiple pregnancies could be reduced or prevented entirely by withholding hCG for patients aged ≤ 32 years, when four or more follicles are ≥ 10 mm in diameter and estradiol concentration is ≥ 862 pg/ml, or when six or more follicles are ≥ 12 mm in diameter for patients aged < 35 years.

In summary, for unknown reasons, singletons conceived after assisted reproduction are significantly disadvantaged compared with naturally conceived singletons. This may not be true for twins, with the possible exception of monozygotic. Nevertheless, pregnancy risk overall is significantly higher for twins, due to the higher rate of multiple pregnancies. Women undergoing assisted reproduction should therefore be informed in detail and in written form of the increased risks in singleton pregnancies, the increased risk of a multiple pregnancy and its inherent risk parameters for both mother and fetuses.

Based on these data, it is clear that infertility treatment faces major challenges to reduce the rate of multiple pregnancies, to consider a multiple pregnancy an adverse outcome of infertility treatment, and to promote techniques aimed at reducing the rate of multiple pregnancies such as single embryo transfer or alternatives to clomiphene stimulation of the ovary.

REFERENCES

1. Navot D, Bergh PA, Laufer N. Ovarian hyperstimulation syndrome in novel reproductive technologies: prevention and treatment. Fertil Steril 1992; 58: 249–61
2. Smits G, Olatunbosun OA, Delbaere A, et al. Spontaneous ovarian hyperstimulation syndrome caused by a mutant follitropin receptor. N Engl J Med 2003; 349: 760–6
3. Golan A, Ron-El R, Herman A, et al. Ovarian hyperstimulation syndrome: an update review. Obstet Gynecol Surv 1989; 44: 430–40
4. Cluroe AD, Synek BJ. A fatal case of ovarian hyperstimulation syndrome with cerebral infarction. Pathology 1995; 27: 344–6
5. Wiser A, Levron J, Kreizer D, et al. Outcome of pregnancies complicated by severe ovarian hyperstimulation syndrome (OHSS): a follow-up beyond the second trimester. Hum Reprod 2005; 20: 910–14
6. Lyons D, Wheeler CA, Frishman GN, et al. Early and late presentation of the ovarian hyperstimulation syndrome: two distinct entities with different risk factors. Hum Reprod 1994; 9: 792–9
7. Beerendonk CC, van Dop PA, Braat DD, Merkus JM. Ovarian hyperstimulation syndrome: facts and fallacies. Obstet Gynecol Surv 1998; 53: 439–49
8. Kol S. Luteolysis induced by a gonadotropin-releasing hormone agonist is the key to prevention of ovarian hyperstimulation syndrome. Fertil Steril 2004; 81: 1–5
9. Orvieto R. Can we eliminate severe ovarian hyperstimulation syndrome? Hum Reprod 2005; 20: 320–2
10. Aboulghar M, Evers JH, Al-Inany H. Intravenous albumin for preventing severe ovarian hyperstimulation syndrome: a Cochrane review. Hum Reprod 2002; 17: 3027–32
11. Wright VC, Schieve LA, Reynolds MA, Jeng G. Assisted reproductive technology surveillance – United States, 2000. MMWR Surveil 2003; 52: 1–16
12. Nyboe Andersen A, Gianaroli L, Nygren KG. European IVF-monitoring programme, European Society of Human Reproduction and Embryology. Assisted reproductive technology in Europe, 2000: results generated from European registers by ESHRE. Hum Reprod 2004; 19: 490–503
13. Blondel B, Kaminski M. Trends in the occurrence, determinants, and consequences of multiple births. Semin Perinatol 2002; 26: 239–49
14. Helmerhorst FM, Perquin DA, Donker D, Keirse MJ. Perinatal outcome of singletons and twins after assisted conception: a systematic review of controlled studies. Br Med J 2004; 328: 261
15. Jackson RA, Gibson KA, Wu YW, Croughan MS. Perinatal outcomes in singletons following in vitro fertilization: a meta-analysis. Obstet Gynecol 2004; 103: 551–63

16. Pinborg A, Loft A, Rasmussen S, et al. Neonatal outcome in a Danish national cohort of 3438 IVF/ICSI and 10,362 non-IVF/ICSI twins born between 1995 and 2000. Hum Reprod 2004; 19: 435–41

17. Verstraelen H, Goetgeluk S, Derom C, et al. Preterm birth in twins after subfertility treatment: population based cohort study. Br Med J 2005; 331: 1173

18. Adashi EY, Rock JA, Sapp KC, et al. Gestational outcome of clomiphene-related conceptions. Fertil Steril 1979; 31: 620–6

19. Dickey RP, Taylor SN, Curole DN, et al. Incidence of spontaneous abortion in clomiphene pregnancies. Hum Reprod 1996; 11: 2623–8

20. Kurachi K, Aono T, Minagawa J, Miyake A. Congenital malformations of newborn infants after clomiphene-induced ovulation. Fertil Steril 1983; 40: 187–9

21. Dickey RP, Taylor SN, Lu PY, et al. Risk factors for high-order multiple pregnancy and multiple birth after controlled ovarian hyperstimulation: results of 4,062 intrauterine insemination cycles. Fertil Steril 2005; 83: 671–83

Index

Illustrations and tables are denoted by **bold** page numbers

INDEX

T - #0018 - 071024 - C0 - 234/156/12 [14] - CB - 9780415384513 - Gloss Lamination